Approaches to Left Atrial Appendage Exclusion

Editors

RANDALL LEE
MOUSSA C. MANSOUR

INTERVENTIONAL CARDIOLOGY CLINICS

www.interventional.theclinics.com

Consulting Editors
SAMIN K. SHARMA
IGOR F. PALACIOS

April 2014 • Volume 3 • Number 2

ELSEVIER

1600 John F. Kennedy Boulevard • Suite 1800 • Philadelphia, Pennsylvania, 19103-2899

http://www.theclinics.com

INTERVENTIONAL CARDIOLOGY CLINICS Volume 3, Number 2
April 2014 ISSN 2211-7458, ISBN-13: 978-0-323-29002-9

Editor: Adrianne Brigido
Developmental Editor: Barbara Cohen-Kligerman

Interventional Cardiology Clinics (ISSN 2211-7458) is published quarterly by Elsevier Inc., 360 Park Avenue South, New York, NY 10010-1710. Months of issue are January, April, July, and October. Subscription prices are USD 195 per year for US individuals, USD 305 for US institutions, USD 130 per year for US students, USD 230 per year for Canadian individuals, USD 375 for Canadian institutions, USD 150 per year for Canadian students, USD 295 per year for international individuals, USD 375 for international institutions, and USD 150 per year for international students. To receive student/resident rate, orders must be accompanied by name of affiliated institution, date of term, and the *signature* of program/residency coordinator on institution letterhead. Orders will be billed at individual rate until proof of status is received. Foreign air speed delivery is included in all *Clinics* subscription prices. All prices are subject to change without notice. **POSTMASTER:** Send address changes to *Interventional Cardiology Clinics*, Elsevier Health Sciences Division, Subscription Customer Service, 3251 Riverport Lane, Maryland Heights, MO 63043. **Customer Service: Telephone: 1-800-654-2452** (U.S. and Canada); **1-314-447-8871** (outside U.S. and Canada). **Fax: 1-314-447-8029. E-mail: journalscustomerservice-usa@elsevier.com** (for print support); **journalsonlinesupport-usa@elsevier.com** (for online support).

Reprints. For copies of 100 or more of articles in this publication, please contact the Commercial Reprints Department, Elsevier Inc., 360 Park Avenue South, New York, NY 10010-1710. Tel.: 212-633-3874; Fax: 212-633-3820; E-mail: reprints@elsevier.com.

Printed and bound by CPI Group (UK) Ltd, Croydon, CR0 4YY

Contributors

CONSULTING EDITORS

SAMIN K. SHARMA, MD, FSCAI, FACC
Director of Clinical Cardiology; Director of
Cardiac Catheterization Laboratory, Mount
Sinai Medical Center, New York, New York

IGOR F. PALACIOS, MD, FSCAI
Director of Interventional Cardiology,
Cardiology Division, Heart Center,
Massachusetts General Hospital; Associate
Professor of Medicine, Harvard Medical
School, Boston, Massachusetts

EDITORS

RANDALL LEE, MD, PhD
Cardiac Electrophysiology, University of
California San Francisco, San Francisco,
California

MOUSSA C. MANSOUR, MD, FHRS, FACC
Massachusetts General Hospital, Cardiac
Arrhythmia Service, Boston, Massachusetts

AUTHORS

RONG BAI, MD
Department of Cardiology, Texas Cardiac
Arrhythmia Institute, St. David's Medical
Center, Austin, Texas

CONOR BARRETT, MD
Department of Cardiology, Al-Sabah
Arrhythmia Institute, St. Luke's Hospital,
New York, New York

J. DAVID BURKHARDT, MD
Department of Cardiology, Texas Cardiac
Arrhythmia Institute, St. David's Medical
Center, Austin, Texas

RALPH J. DAMIANO Jr, MD
John M. Shoenberg Professor of Surgery; Chief
of Cardiac Surgery, Division of Cardiothoracic
Surgery, Barnes-Jewish Hospital, Washington
University School of Medicine, St Louis,
Missouri

STEPHAN DANIK, MD
Department of Cardiology, Al-Sabah
Arrhythmia Institute, St. Luke's Hospital,
New York, New York

BUDDHADEB DAWN, MD
Maureen and Marvin Dunn Professor; Director,
Division of Cardiovascular Diseases; Director,
Cardiovascular Research Institute; Director,
Midwest Stem Cell Therapy Center; Vice
Chairman for Research, Department of
Medicine, Division of Cardiovascular Medicine,
Mid-America Cardiology, University of Kansas
Hospital, University of Kansas Medical Center,
Kansas City, Kansas

LUIGI DI BIASE, MD, PhD
Department of Cardiology, University of
Foggia, Foggia, Italy; Department of
Cardiology, Texas Cardiac Arrhythmia
Institute, St. David's Medical Center, Austin,
Texas; Division of Cardiology, Montefiore
Hospital, Albert Einstein College of Medicine,
Bronx, New York; Department of Biomedical
Engineering, University of Texas, Austin,
Texas

DAVID M. DUDZINSKI, MD, JD
Echocardiography Laboratory; Cardiology
Division, Massachusetts General Hospital,
Boston, Massachusetts

MATTHEW B. EARNEST, MD, FACC, FSCAI
Clinical Assistant Professor of Medicine,
Medical Director of Chest Pain Services,
Mid-America Cardiology, University of Kansas
Hospital, Kansas City, Kansas

TED FELDMAN, MD, FESC, FACC, FSCAI
Cardiology Division, Evanston Hospital,
NorthShore University HealthSystem,
Evanston, Illinois

RYAN FERRELL, MD, FACC, FACP
Associate Professor, Cardiovascular Diseases,
Division of Cardiovascular Medicine,
Mid-America Cardiology, University of
Kansas Hospital, University of Kansas
Medical Center, Kansas City, Kansas

E. KEVIN HEIST, MD, PhD
Associate Professor of Medicine, Harvard
Medical School; Cardiac Arrhythmia Service,
Massachusetts General Hospital, Boston,
Massachusetts

RODNEY HORTON, MD
Department of Cardiology, Texas Cardiac
Arrhythmia Institute, St. David's Medical
Center, Austin, Texas

JUDY HUNG, MD
Associate Director, Echocardiography;
Associate Professor of Medicine, Cardiology
Division, Massachusetts General Hospital,
Harvard Medical School, Boston,
Massachusetts

ARUN KANMANTHAREDDY, MD, MS
Fellow, Division of Cardiovascular Medicine,
Mid-America Cardiology, University of Kansas
Hospital, University of Kansas Medical Center,
Kansas City, Kansas

SAIBAL KAR, MD, FACC
Director of Interventional Cardiac Research,
Heart Institute, Cedars-Sinai Medical Center;
David Geffen School of Medicine at University
of California, Los Angeles, Los Angeles,
California

**DHANUNJAYA LAKKIREDDY, MD, FACC,
FHRS**
Professor of Medicine, Division of Cardiology,
Mid-America Cardiology; Director, Center
for Excellence in Atrial Fibrillation and
Electrophysiology Research, Bloch Heart
Rhythm Center, KU Cardiovascular Research
Institute, University of Kansas Hospital,
University of Kansas Medical Center, Kansas
City, Kansas

ABHISHEK MAAN, MD
Research Fellow, Harvard Medical School;
Cardiac Arrhythmia Service, Massachusetts
General Hospital, Boston, Massachusetts

ALESSANDRO MONTECALVO, MD
Division of Cardiothoracic Surgery,
Barnes-Jewish Hospital, Washington
University School of Medicine, St Louis,
Missouri

ANDREA NATALE, MD
Department of Cardiology, Texas Cardiac
Arrhythmia Institute, St. David's Medical
Center; Department of Biomedical Engineering,
University of Texas, Austin, Texas; EP
Services, California Pacific Medical Center,
San Francisco; Division of Cardiology,
Stanford University, Stanford, California;
Division of Cardiovascular Medicine, Case
Western Reserve University, University
Hospitals of Cleveland, Cleveland, Ohio;
Interventional Electrophysiology, Department
of Cardiology, Scripps Clinic, La Jolla,
California

JAYANT NATH, MD
Division of Cardiovascular Medicine,
Mid-America Cardiology, University of Kansas
Hospital, University of Kansas Medical Center,
Kansas City, Kansas

MATTHEW J. PRICE, MD, FACC, FSCAI
Division of Cardiovascular Diseases, Scripps
Clinic and Scripps Translational Science
Institute, La Jolla, California

YERUVA MADHU REDDY, MD
Assistant Professor of Medicine, Division
of Cardiovascular Medicine, University of
Kansas Hospital, Kansas City, Kansas

JEREMY N. RUSKIN, MD
Associate Professor of Medicine, Harvard
Medical School; Cardiac Arrhythmia Service,
Massachusetts General Hospital, Boston,
Massachusetts

PASQUALE SANTANGELI, MD
Department of Cardiology, University of Foggia, Foggia, Italy; Department of Cardiology, Texas Cardiac Arrhythmia Institute, St. David's Medical Center, Austin, Texas

FRANCESCO SANTORO, MD
Department of Cardiology, University of Foggia, Foggia, Italy

SHMUEL SCHWARTZENBERG, MD
Echocardiography Laboratory; Cardiology Division, Massachusetts General Hospital, Boston, Massachusetts

ZOLTAN G. TURI, MD
Director, Structural Heart Disease Program; Professor of Medicine, Department of Medicine, Rutgers Robert Wood Johnson Medical School, New Brunswick, New Jersey

GAURAV A. UPADHYAY, MD
Cardiac Electrophysiology Division; Cardiology Division, Massachusetts General Hospital, Boston, Massachusetts

MIGUEL VALDERRÁBANO, MD
Director, Division of Cardiac Electrophysiology, Department of Cardiology, Methodist DeBakey Heart and Vascular Center, Houston Methodist Hospital; Adjunct Associate Professor of Medicine, Baylor College of Medicine; Associate Professor of Medicine, Weill College of Medicine, Cornell University, Houston, Texas

AJAY VALLAKATI, MD
Division of Cardiology, Metro Health Medical Center, Case Western Reserve University, Cleveland, Ohio

PETER WEISS, MD
Division of Cardiology, Intermountain Medical Center, Salt Lake City, Utah

BRIAN WHISENANT, MD
Division of Cardiology, Intermountain Medical Center, Salt Lake City, Utah

WEN-LOONG YEOW, MD
Heart Institute, Cedars-Sinai Medical Center, Los Angeles, California

Contents

Stroke and Bleeding Risks in Patients with Atrial Fibrillation   175

Abhishek Maan, Jeremy N. Ruskin, and E. Kevin Heist

Atrial fibrillation (AF) is the most common cardiac arrhythmia and is associated with a substantial risk of stroke and mortality. Strokes in patients with AF are associated with a greater disability and poorer outcomes than strokes in patients in sinus rhythm. Patients with AF are at increased risk of bleeding, especially if they use anticoagulant therapy. Recent research in the field of anticoagulation has led to development of new anticoagulants for stroke prevention in addition to antiplatelet agents and warfarin. This review discusses the role of AF as a risk factor for stroke and evaluates the role of various schemes for predicting the risk of stroke and bleeding in patients with AF.

Embryology and Anatomy of the Left Atrial Appendage: Why Does Thrombus Form?   191

Arun Kanmanthareddy, Yeruva Madhu Reddy, Ajay Vallakati, Matthew B. Earnest, Jayant Nath, Ryan Ferrell, Buddhadeb Dawn, and Dhanunjaya Lakkireddy

The left atrial appendage (LAA) is a long tubular structure that opens into the left atrium. In patients with atrial fibrillation, the LAA develops mechanical dysfunction and fibroelastotic changes on the endocardial surface. The complex anatomy of the LAA makes it a good site for relative blood stasis. In addition, systemic factors exacerbate the hypercoagulable state, eventually resulting in endothelial dysfunction, release of tissue factor, and production of inflammatory cytokines and oxidative free radicals, and eventually initiating the coagulation cascade. Thus, the LAA is susceptible to thrombus formation and is the most common source of systemic thromboembolism.

Rationale for Left Atrial Appendage Exclusion   203

Ted Feldman

Left atrial appendage (LAA) is the source of most systemic emboli in patients with atrial fibrillation. Oral anticoagulant therapy reduces stroke risk by two-thirds. New oral agents have advantages over warfarin but are associated with bleeding and drug intolerance. Device therapy for atrial appendage ligation or occlusion is an alternative to drug therapy, without the cumulative incidence of bleeding or the need for anticoagulation. In the more than half century since the early reports of surgical LAA excision, the author has added considerable detail to our understanding of the rationale for LAA exclusion, which constitutes the subject of this article.

Left Atrial Appendage Closure with Transcatheter-Delivered Devices   209

Brian Whisenant and Peter Weiss

Left atrial appendage (LAA) closure with transcatheter-delivered devices is an evolving story of compelling randomized data and the potential to dramatically reduce the incidence of stroke and improve the quality of life among patients with atrial fibrillation. Oral anticoagulation is the standard of care for stroke prevention

INTERVENTIONAL CARDIOLOGY CLINICS

Preface
Approaches to Left Atrial Appendage Exclusion

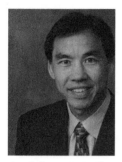 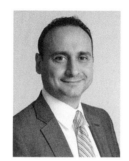

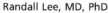

Randall Lee, MD, PhD   Moussa C. Mansour, MD, FHRS, FACC
Editors

Atrial fibrillation is currently the most prevalent arrhythmia in the United States, and its prevalence is projected to increase significantly. The most severe consequence of atrial fibrillation is cardioembolic stroke. The mainstay of the prevention of stroke has been warfarin therapy. However, due to the difficulty of maintaining adequate anticoagulation levels, multiple interactions with food and other medications, and the risk of bleeding events, alternative therapies have been established. Despite the development of newer oral anticoagulation agents, problems with side effects, compliance, and bleeding still occur.

The left atrial appendage is a prominent source of cardioembolic stroke in patients with nonvalvular atrial fibrillation. This issue of *Interventional Cardiology Clinics* is dedicated to the role of catheter-based left atrial closure for the treatment of patients with nonvalvular atrial fibrillation who are at risk for cardioembolic events. Articles in this issue provide an overview of the magnitude of the problem of stroke in patients with atrial fibrillation, the role of the left atrial appendage in thrombus formation, and the rationale for exclusion of the left atrial appendage with devices. Different approaches for excluding the left atrial appendage, tips and tricks for successful left atrial

appendage exclusion, and review of the clinical evidence for percutaneous left atrial appendage exclusion are discussed. Special attention is paid to the use of transesophageal echocardiography and how to obtain pericardial access as part of the procedure in performing left atrial appendage closure. Finally, a section is dedicated to prevention and management of complications. The editors would like to thank all the authors who contributed to this comprehensive overview of device therapy for left atrial appendage exclusion.

Randall Lee, MD, PhD
Cardiac Electrophysiology
University of California San Francisco
Box 1354, 500 Parnassus Avenue
San Francisco, CA 94143-1354, USA

Moussa C. Mansour, MD, FHRS, FACC
Massachusetts General Hospital
Cardiac Arrhythmia Service, GRB 109
55 Fruit Street
Boston, MA 02114, USA

E-mail addresses:
Lee@medicine.ucsf.edu (R. Lee)
mmansour@partners.org (M.C. Mansour)

Intervent Cardiol Clin 3 (2014) xi
http://dx.doi.org/10.1016/j.iccl.2014.02.001
2211-7458/14/$ – see front matter © 2014 Published by Elsevier Inc.

Stroke and Bleeding Risks in Patients with Atrial Fibrillation

Abhishek Maan, MD, Jeremy N. Ruskin, MD,
E. Kevin Heist, MD, PhD*

KEYWORDS

• Atrial fibrillation • Anticoagulant therapy • Stroke

KEY POINTS

• Atrial fibrillation (AF) is associated with a substantially increased risk of thromboembolic stroke.
• Antiplatelet agents have some effect in reducing the stroke risk associated with AF but are less effective than anticoagulants, such as warfarin, in this regard.
• Newer oral anticoagulants (OACs)—dabigatran, rivaroxaban, and apixaban—are at least as effective as warfarin in reducing AF-associated stroke.
• Anticoagulants used for stroke prevention in AF cause an increased risk of bleeding. Scoring systems are available to better estimate an individual patient's bleeding risk.

INTRODUCTION

AF is the most common cardiac arrhythmia encountered in clinical practice.[1] The presence of this arrhythmia is an independent risk factor for stroke/thromboembolism and death, with an estimated 5-fold higher risk.[2,3] Anticoagulation with OACs and antiplatelet agents is the mainstay for stroke prophylaxis in patients with AF. A meta-analysis by Hart and colleagues[4] demonstrated that dose-adjusted warfarin resulted in 64% reduction of stroke and a 26% reduction in all-cause mortality compared with placebo, and antiplatelet therapy resulted in 22% reduction in stroke with no significant reduction in mortality. Recent conclusion of major clinical trials has led to the Food and Drug Administration approval of newer OACs, which has expanded the armamentarium of anticoagulation options for stroke prophylaxis in patients with AF.

Stroke risk is closely related to bleeding risk in AF patients.[5] Many risk factors for thromboembolism, such as advanced age, uncontrolled hypertension, ischemic heart disease, and cerebrovascular disease, have also been identified as risk factors for bleeding.[6,7] Bleeding risk is especially higher with the use of vitamin K antagonists (VKAs) due to their narrow therapeutic window and drug-drug and drug-food interactions.[8] This article reviews the risk of stroke and various risk-prediction schemes to predict stroke risk and bleeding complications in patients with AF and evaluates the role of OACs and antiplatelet agents for stroke prevention.

Dr E.K. Heist is the senior author in this article.
Disclosures: A. Maan: None; J.N. Ruskin: Astellas/Cardiome–consultant (significant), Biosense Webster–consultant (modest) and fellowship support (significant), Boston Scientific–fellowship support (significant), CardioFocus–clinical oversight committee (no compensation), CardioInsight–scientific advisory board (modest), CryoCath–scientific steering committee (no compensation), Medtronic–consultant (modest) and fellowship support (significant), Med-IQ–honoraria (modest), Pfizer–consultant and scientific steering committee (modest), Portola–consultant and equity (modest), Sanofi–consultant (modest), St. Jude Medical–fellowship support (significant), and Third Rock Ventures–consultant (significant); E.K. Heist (all modest in amount): Biotronik (research grant, honoraria), Boston Scientific (research grant, consultant, honoraria), Medtronic (honoraria), Sanofi (consultant), Sorin (consultant, honoraria), and St. Jude Medical (research grant, consultant, honoraria).
Cardiac Arrhythmia Service, Massachusetts General Hospital, 55 Fruit Street, Boston, MA 02114, USA
* Corresponding author.
E-mail address: kheist@partners.org

Intervent Cardiol Clin 3 (2014) 175–190
http://dx.doi.org/10.1016/j.iccl.2013.11.001
2211-7458/14/$ – see front matter © 2014 Elsevier Inc. All rights reserved.

interventional.theclinics.com

METHODS

The authors performed a comprehensive literature search in the PubMed database using the MeSH terms, "atrial fibrillation," "cerebrovascular events," "bleeding complications," and "oral anticoagulants." Original studies and clinical trials describing the epidemiology of AF and risk of stroke in patients with AF and comparing various OAC options for stroke prophylaxis were included.

Stroke Risk in Atrial Fibrillation

AF is an independent risk factor for the risk of stroke. The presence of AF leads to an impaired left atrial contraction, which creates a hypercoagulable state as part of the Virchow triad[9] and is further supported by studies that have demonstrated increased levels of coagulation markers (fibrinogen, D dimer, and fibrinopeptide).[10,11] The effect of this hypercoagulable state is further increased by the endothelial dysfunction[12] and platelet activation.[13,14] With the increased use of device-based therapy for various indications, even transient AF is being investigated as an important risk factor for cryptogenic stroke.[15,16]

Stroke Risk–Prediction Schemes

Various risk-prediction schemes have been developed to estimate the risk of stroke in patients with AF. CHADS$_2$ (congestive heart failure, 1 point; hypertension, 1 point; age >75 years, 1 point; diabetes mellitus, 1 point; and prior history of stroke/transient ischemic attack [TIA], 2 points) is the most commonly used risk-prediction scheme.[17,18] The CHADS$_2$ risk score is essentially derived from the risk factors identified from the non-VKA arms of the stroke prevention trial cohorts and the Framingham study and, due to lack of systemic documentation, many potential risk factors have not been adequately assessed. Another important limitation of the CHADS$_2$ risk scheme is that it has a tendency to classify a proportion of patients as at intermediate risk, thereby including some patients who might be at low risk of thromboembolism.[19]

The CHADS$_2$ score has also been believed to underestimate the effect of age as an important risk factor for stroke. Stroke risk in patients with AF increases from age 65 years upward, and, given that age is a strong predictor for stroke and mortality in AF, it seems that accounting 1 point for all age groups >75 years categorizes older patients with low-risk younger patients, leading to suboptimal thromboprophylaxis in older patients with a CHADS$_2$ score of 1 who are likely to benefit more from OAC therapy.[20]

Vascular disease is another major risk factor for stroke and mortality in patients with AF.[21,22] In the Loire Valley Atrial Fibrillation Project, vascular disease increased the risk of thromboembolism and, along with the CHADS$_2$ score, it improved the predictive ability for stroke.[23] The CHA$_2$DS$_2$-VASc (congestive heart failure, 1 point; hypertension, 1 point; age <65 years, 0 point; age 65–75 years, 1 point; age ≥75 years, 2 points; diabetes, 1 point; stroke/TIA/Thromboembolism, 2 points; vascular disease history, 1 point; Sex: Male, 0 point; Female, 1 point) score was introduced to include the impact of vascular disease and to appropriately account for the effect of age as an important risk factor for stroke; to further complement the CHADS$_2$ score, the new European Society of Cardiology (ESC) guidelines have placed more emphasis on a risk factor–based approach compared with a low-, moderate-, and high-risk stratification. This risk factor–based approach advocated by the ESC tries to be more inclusive rather than exclusive of the common and important risk factors for stroke.[24] This approach is believed to have 2 important advantages: to identify the truly very-low-risk AF patients who do not need antithrombotic therapy and to identify the patients with 1 or more risk factors for stroke who can benefit from the highly effective OAC-based therapy for stroke prophylaxis (**Box 1**).[25]

von Willebrand Factor Levels as a Risk Factor for Stroke

von Willebrand Factor (vWF) has an essential role in hemostasis by promoting platelet adhesion

---

Box 1
Advantages and disadvantages of the CHADS$_2$ score for prediction of stroke risk in patients with AF

Advantages

- Simple and widely applicable
- Identifies low-risk patients in whom the risk of warfarin therapy is greater than the benefit and for whom aspirin may be a reasonable option for stroke prophylaxis
- Well validated

Disadvantages

- Tendency to classify a proportion of low-risk patients as intermediate-risk
- Does not account of risk factors for stroke, such as vascular disease, female gender, vWF, and impaired left ventricular systolic function
- Limited in applicability with the advent of newer OACs

and aggregation, by mediating endothelial dysfunction at the site of vascular injury, and as a carrier protein for factor VIII.[26-28] The role of vWF has also been well investigated in the setting of AF, where elevated levels of vWF have been found associated with abnormal thrombogenesis and intracardiac thrombus.[28,29]

In a prospective study by Wieberdink and colleagues,[30] 6250 patients were followed over a period of 5 years and patients with an elevated level of vWF at baseline were found to have an elevated risk of stroke (age- and gender-adjusted hazard ratios [HRs] per SD increase in vWF level: 1.12 [95% CI, 1.01–1.25]). Considering its key role in endothelial dysfunction and associated risk of stroke in patients with AF, the additive role of plasma levels of vWF to the $CHADS_2$ risk-prediction scheme was investigated on the 994 AF patients who were enrolled in the Stroke Prevention in Atrial Fibrillation (SPAF)-III trial.[31] These patients were originally classified into low-, moderate-, and high-risk categories according to the Birmingham[32] and $CHADS_2$ risk-prediction schemes (**Fig. 1**). vWF levels were categorized as elevated at greater than 158 IU/dL and, when added to the Birmingham risk-prediction scheme, elevated plasma levels of vWF were independently associated with an increased risk of vascular events (HR 2.06; 95% CI, 1.30–3.22); when added to the $CHADS_2$ risk-prediction scheme, elevated plasma levels of vWF were independently associated with the risk of vascular events (HR 2.01; 95% CI, 1.27–3.18).[33] The measurement of plasma levels of vWF and its addition to the risk-prediction schemes can be especially useful in moderate-risk patients in whom current treatment guidelines are not clear about the use of either warfarin or aspirin for stroke prophylaxis.

AF Burden as a Risk Factor for Stroke

With the recent increase in the use of device therapy for various clinical indications in AF patients, the role of AF burden as an important risk factor for stroke has emerged as another newer area of investigation. Because AF burden can now be measured with an increased accuracy, it is reasonable to intuitively associate a greater degree of AF burden with an increased risk of cerebrovascular events.

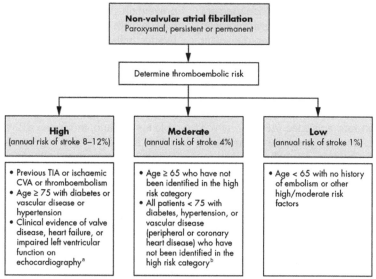

Fig. 1. Birmingham risk stratification for prediction of stroke risk in patients with AF. The risk factors described are not mutually exclusive but additive in nature. Note that risk factors are not mutually exclusive and are additive to each other in producing a composite risk. [a] An echocardiogram is not needed for routine risk assessment but refines clinical risk stratification in case of moderate or severe left ventricular dysfunction and valve disease. Because the incidence of thromboembolic events in patients with thyrotoxicosis appears similar to that of other etiologies of AF, antithrombotic therapies should be chosen on the basis of the presence of validated stroke risk factors. [b] Owing to a lack of sufficient clearcut evidence, risk assessment may be decided on an individual basis, and physicians must balance the risks and benefits of warfarin versus aspirin; because stroke risk factors are cumulative, warfarin may, for example, be used in the presence of 2 or more risk factors. Referral and echocardiography may help in cases of uncertainty. CVA, cerebrovascular accident. (*From* Lip GY, Lane D, Van Walraven C, et al. Additive role of plasma von Willebrand factor levels to clinical factors for risk stratification of patients with atrial fibrillation. Stroke 2006;37:2295; with permission.)

In the Copenhagen City Heart Study, elevated levels of fibrinogen were associated with an increased risk of AF after adjusting for other cardiovascular risk factors[34]; because fibrinogen is a key mediator of thrombogenesis, its elevated levels in AF patients further support the role of AF in thrombogenesis. In another study by Sohara and colleagues,[35] the patients with paroxysmal AF were found to have elevated levels of P-selectin within 12 hours of arrhythmia onset, and the increased levels of P-selectin persisted for a longer duration in patients who had more sustained type of AF. Although it is fairly clear that various biomarkers mediating endothelial dysfunction, platelet activation, and thrombogenesis are significantly elevated in patients with AF compared with sinus rhythm, studies investigating the temporal patterns of AF and biomarker levels are limited and have shown variable results.

Also, the limitations of the current classification of chronologic subtypes of AF in terms of predicting the risk of stroke and thromboembolism become especially important in the setting of a substantial proportion of patients having had asymptomatic AF for a long time and tending to present with stroke or systemic embolism for the first time. In an analysis of the Atrial Fibrillation Follow-up Investigation of Rhythm Management (AFFIRM) study, patients who had asymptomatic AF had a higher incidence of cerebrovascular events and received fewer cardioprotective medications compared with patients who were symptomatic at baseline.[36] The advent and increased use of device therapy in patients with AF also offers the advantage of characterization and measurement of atrial high-rate episodes (AHREs), which has emerged as another predictor of adverse events in these patients. In a substudy based on 312 patients from the Mode Selection Trial (MOST) trial, patients who had at least 1 episode of AHRE of greater than 5 minutes' duration had a 5.93-fold higher risk of developing AF and 2.79-fold higher risk of death or nonfatal stroke.[37] Further studies will help clarify the role of AHREs as a risk factor for stroke and thromboembolism.

Antiplatelet Therapy for Stroke Prevention in AF

A meta-analysis of 8 randomized trials by Hart and colleagues[4] reported that antiplatelet therapy reduced the risk of stroke in patients with AF by 22% compared with placebo; when this analysis was confined to the aspirin-only clinical trials (n = 3990 across 7 clinical trials), stroke was reduced by 19% (95% CI, −1 to 35) and the mortality risk was also reduced by 14% (95% CI, −7 to 31); however, these risk reductions were not statistically significant. In these clinical trials, the dose of aspirin varied widely from 50 to 1300 mg per day. The Copenhagen Atrial Fibrillation, Aspirin, and Anticoagulation (AFASAK) study was one of the earliest studies to demonstrate the protective role of warfarin and aspirin for stroke prophylaxis in patients with AF.[38] In the SPAF-I trial, there was an overall 42% reduction in the rate of primary events (ischemic stroke and systemic embolism) with the use of 325-mg daily dose of aspirin compared with placebo (6.3% per year in the placebo arm vs 3.6% per year in the aspirin arm; $P = .02$; 95% CI, 9%–63%) based on the pooled results from the anticoagulation-eligible and anticoagulation-ineligible arms; also, the risk reduction in stroke with the use of aspirin was heterogeneous 94% risk reduction ($P<.001$) in the anticoagulation-eligible and 8% in the anticoagulation-ineligible patients ($P = .75$). Aspirin was also ineffective in patients older than 75 years of age and did not prevent severe strokes[39]; also, the exclusion of high-risk patients (patients with recent stroke and systemic embolism) from the SPAF-I trial could have led to the enhanced effect of aspirin. Combination antiplatelet therapy has also been investigated for stroke prevention in AF in the Atrial Fibrillation Clopidogrel Trial with Irbesartan for Prevention of Vascular Events trials (ACTIVE W and ACTIVE A).[40,41] In the ACTIVE W trial, OAC was superior to the combination of aspirin and clopidogrel for the prevention of stroke and vascular events in the patients with AF.[40] In the ACTIVE A trial, which included AF patients at high risk of stroke who were unsuitable for warfarin, there was a 28% reduction in the risk of stroke with the combination of aspirin and clopidogrel compared with aspirin alone.[41]

Antiplatelet therapy has also been investigated in combination with VKAs to assess whether the combination therapy enabled the intensity of anticoagulation to be decreased to reduce the risk of excessive bleeding without reducing the primary efficacy for prevention of stroke in patients with AF. The SPAF-III trial compared aspirin and fixed-dose warfarin (to maintain an international normalized ratio [INR] 1.2–1.5) with adjusted-dose warfarin (to maintain an INR 2.0–3.0) in patients with nonvalvular AF at high risk of thromboembolism. There was a significantly higher number of ischemic stroke and systemic embolism in the combination group of aspirin and fixed-dose warfarin compared with the warfarin-alone group ($P<.001$); hence, the trial had to be stopped earlier than the anticipated date.[31] In light of these findings, the Second Copenhagen Atrial Fibrillation, Aspirin, and Anticoagulation (AFASAK

2) study, assessing the efficacy and safety of fixed low-dose warfarin with (or without aspirin) compared with aspirin or dose-adjusted warfarin, was also stopped earlier than the anticipated completion date.[42] The clinical trials investigating the role of antiplatelet therapy for stroke prevention in patients with AF are summarized in **Table 1**.

These results demonstrating the efficacy of antiplatelet therapy imply that platelets could play some (although limited) role in the pathogenesis of stroke in patients with AF. This efficacy could, however, be predominantly attributed to the inhibition of platelet thrombi in the carotid and cerebral arteries than the thrombi that occur as a direct result of AF.[43] There are certain pathophysiologic considerations that should be kept in mind, such as that platelet dysfunction and complex atherosclerotic plaques are common coexisting conditions in many patients with AF[44,45] and thus the effect of antiplatelet therapy could also be mediated by the regression of atherosclerotic vascular disease; also it has been well-proved that the thrombi in vascular disease are platelet rich (white clot) and, therefore, respond to antiplatelet therapy, whereas the thrombi in AF are fibrin rich (red clot) and, therefore, respond to the anticoagulant therapy.[45]

Warfarin for Stroke Prophylaxis in Patients with AF

Warfarin has been the most extensively evaluated OAC for the prevention of stroke in patients with AF. SPAF-I was one of the major multicentric trials that demonstrated that a dose-adjusted warfarin was 67% effective in reducing the risk of ischemic stroke and systemic embolism compared with placebo (2.3% in the warfarin arm vs 7.4% in the placebo arm; $P = .01$); warfarin was also shown to have mortality benefit compared with placebo and aspirin in the patients with AF who were at increased risk of stroke.[38] Similar results in favor of warfarin for stroke prevention were also reported in the Copenhagen AFASAK and the Canadian Atrial Fibrillation Anticoagulation (CAFA) studies.[39,46] The results of various clinical trials demonstrating the efficacy of warfarin for stroke prophylaxis are summarized in **Table 2**.

Despite the clear benefit of warfarin for the prevention of stroke and the clinical experience with the use of warfarin, the limitations of warfarin have also posed a major challenge in routine clinical practice. Warfarin has multiple drug-drug and drug-food interactions that make its use in patients with AF particularly challenging because these patients are also taking other medications due to

Table 1
Rate of stroke, systemic embolism, and bleeding in clinical trials investigating dual antiplatelet therapy in patients with nonvalvular AF

Study	Population	Treatment Groups	Efficacy and Safety End Points	Incidence of Efficacy End Point	Incidence of Safety End Point
ACTIVE W[a,40]	6706 AF patients with ≥1 risk factors	a. VKA (INR 2–3) or b. Aspirin (75–100 mg/d) + clopidogrel (75 mg/d)	Stroke, non-CNS systemic embolism, MI, vascular death Safety Safety: major bleeding	3.93% In the VKA arm vs 5.60% in the (aspirin + clopidogrel) arm	2.21% In the VKA arm vs 2.425 in the aspirin + clopidogrel arm
ACTIVE A[41]	7554 AF patients unsuitable for VKA therapy	a. Aspirin (75–100 mg/d) + clopidogrel (75 mg/d) or b. Aspirin (75–100 mg/d) + placebo	Same as ACTIVE W	6.8% In the (aspirin + clopidogrel) arm vs 7.6% in the (aspirin + placebo) arm	2.0% In the (aspirin + clopidogrel) arm vs 1.3% in the (aspirin + placebo) arm

Risk factors: age ≥75 years, hypertension, previous stroke/TIA, non-CNS systemic embolism, ejection fraction <45%, peripheral arterial disease, or age 55–74 years with diabetes or previous coronary artery disease. The ACTIVE A trial included patients who were not suitable for VKA therapy.

Abbreviations: CNS, central nervous system; MI, myocardial infarction.

[a] ACTIVE W: Clopidogrel plus aspirin versus oral anticoagulation for atrial fibrillation in the Atrial fibrillation Clopidogrel Trial with Irbesartan for prevention of Vascular Events (ACTIVE W). In the ACTIVE W trial of the ACTIVE programme, the patients who were eligible for and willing to take oral anticoagulation were enrolled, in this trial a combination of aspirin + clopidogrel was compared to oral anticoagulation therapy.

Table 2
Rates of stroke, systemic embolism, and bleeding in clinical trials investigating warfarin in patients with nonvalvular atrial fibrillation

Study	Treatment Groups	Efficacy and Safety End Points	Annual Risk of Efficacy End Points	Annual Risk of Safety End Points
AFASAK[38]	a. Warfarin (adjusted dose) b. Aspirin 75 mg/d, placebo	Efficacy: thromboembolic phenomenon (TIA, stroke, embolism to viscera and extremities) Safety: bleeding events	2.0% In the warfarin arm vs 5.5% in the aspirin arm	6.27% In the warfarin arm vs 0.60% in the aspirin arm
SPAF-I[39]	a. Warfarin (adjusted dose) vs placebo vs b. Aspirin 325 mg/d compared with placebo	Efficacy: ischemic stroke and systemic embolism Safety: bleeding events	2.3% In the warfarin arm, 3.6% in the aspirin arm 7.4% And 6.3% in the placebo arms, respectively	1.5% In the warfarin arm vs 1.4% in the aspirin arm and 1.6% in the placebo arm
SPAF-III[31]	a. Fixed-dose warfarin (INR 1.2–1.5) + aspirin 325 mg/d vs b. Adjusted-dose warfarin (INR 2.0–3.0)	Efficacy: ischemic stroke and systemic embolism Safety: major hemorrhage	7.9% In the fixed-dose warfarin + aspirin arm vs 1.9% in the adjusted-dose warfarin arm	2.4% In the fixed-dose warfarin + aspirin arm vs 2.1% in the adjusted-dose warfarin arm
AFASAK-2[42]	a. Minidose warfarin (1.25 mg/d) b. Warfarin (1.25 mg/d) + aspirin 300 mg/d c. Aspirin 300 mg/d d. Adjusted-dose warfarin (INR 2.0–3.0)	Efficacy: ischemic stroke and systemic embolism Safety: major hemorrhage	5.8% In the minidose warfarin arm, 7.2% in the minidose warfarin + aspirin arm, 3.6% in the aspirin arm, 2.8% in the adjusted-dose warfarin arm	8.23% In minidose warfarin arm, 8.13% in the minidose warfarin + aspirin arm, 10% in the aspirin arm, 13.7% in the adjusted-dose warfarin arm
CAFA[46]	a. Warfarin vs b. Placebo	Efficacy: ischemic stroke and systemic embolism Safety: bleeding events	3.5% In the warfarin arm vs 5.2% in the placebo arm	2.5% In the warfarin arm vs 0.5% in the placebo arm

their coexisting cardiovascular conditions. The use of warfarin is also limited by the inter- and intraindividual variations in the efficacy of warfarin, highlighted by the wide variations in the time in therapeutic-range INR spent by the patients in the warfarin arm of various clinical trials. These limitations have led to the emergence of novel OACs for the purpose of stroke prophylaxis in the patients with AF.

Novel OACs and the Risk of Stroke in Patients with AF

The Randomized Evaluation of Long-Term Anticoagulation Therapy (RE-LY) was the first major multicentric randomized clinical trial (RCT) that compared a dose-adjusted warfarin with 2 different doses of dabigatran (110 mg and 150 mg twice daily, each administered in a blinded manner in two different arms); the rate of stroke and systemic embolism was 1.69% per year in the warfarin arm compared with 1.53% per year in the arm that received 110-mg of dabigatran and 1.11% per year in the 150-mg dabigatran arm ($P<.001$ for noninferiority).[47] Similar results demonstrating the efficacy of rivaroxaban for the prevention of stroke in patients with AF were also reported in the Rivaroxaban Once-Daily Oral Direct Factor Xa Inhibition Compared with Vitamin K Antagonism for Prevention of Stroke and

Embolism Trial in Atrial Fibrillation (ROCKET-AF) trial. The incidence of primary efficacy outcomes (composite of stroke and systemic embolism) was 1.7% per year in the rivaroxaban compared with 2.2% per year in the warfarin arm demonstrating the noninferiority of rivaroxaban for the prevention of stroke in patients with AF.[48] The Apixaban for Reduction of Stroke and Other Thromboembolic Events in Atrial Fibrillation (ARISTOTLE) trial was the latest trial, which also demonstrated that apixaban was noninferior to warfarin for the prevention of stroke. The incidence of stroke and systemic embolism was 1.27% per year in the apixaban group compared with 1.60% per year in the warfarin group (*P*<.001 for noninferiority).[49] The incidence of stroke, systemic embolism, and hemorrhagic stroke with the use of newer OACs in comparison with warfarin in these clinical trials is summarized in **Table 3**.

Bleeding Risk

The results of various clinical trials and experience based on the use of OACs in the routine clinical practice has led to the emergence of anticoagulant therapy as the mainstay for the prevention of stroke in patients with AF; however, bleeding remains the major complication of OAC therapy that leads to lack or underprescription of OACs in patients.[50,51] In patients with AF, the risk of stroke is also closely related to the risk of bleeding[4,52]; many risk factors, such as older

age, uncontrolled hypertension, coronary artery disease, diabetes, and cerebrovascular disease, have been identified as common risk factors for both bleeding and thromboembolic events.[5,6] Advanced age has been shown an important common risk factor for not only increased incidence of bleeding but also intracranial bleeding in various studies; this effect of age has been speculated due to the presence of coexisting cardiovascular and peripheral vascular disease in this population.[4,52] A study by Fang and colleagues[53] identified that the rate of bleeding in patients older than 85 years of age was particularly high with an INR greater than 3.5; however, intracranial hemorrhage did also occur with subtherapeutic INR. These findings seem to support the role of various INR-independent pathways responsible for bleeding in this population. Elderly patients have a higher prevalence of microvascular dysfunction, leukoaraiosis, and cerebral amyloid angiopathy, which could have led to increased incidence of intracerebral hemorrhage.[54,55]

Bleeding Risk Definition in Major Clinical Trials

The majority of RCTs have used International Society on Thrombosis and Haemostasis (ISTH) criteria for major bleeding,[56] which classifies fatal bleeding and/or overt bleeding with a drop in hemoglobin level of at least 20 g/L or requiring transfusion of at least 2 units of packed blood cells, or hemorrhage into a critical anatomic site (eg,

---

Table 3
Rate of stroke, systemic embolism, and bleeding in clinical trials investigating newer oral anticoagulants versus warfarin in patients with nonvalvular atrial fibrillation

Study	Treatment Groups	Efficacy and Safety End Points	Annual Risk of Efficacy Outcome	Annual Risk of Safety Outcome
RE-LY[47]	Warfarin (INR 2.0–3.0) vs dabigatran 150 mg, 110 mg bid	Stroke or systemic embolism	1.69% In the warfarin arm vs 1.11% in dabigatran 150 mg, 1.53% dabigatran 110 mg arm	3.36% In the warfarin arm vs 3.11% in dabigatran 150 mg, 2.71% dabigatran 110 mg arm
ROCKET-AF[48]	Warfarin (INR 2.0–3.0) vs rivaroxaban 20 mg daily [a]	Stroke or systemic embolism, major bleeding or clinically relevant nonmajor bleeding	2.2% In the warfarin arm vs 1.7% in rivaroxaban arm	14.5% In the warfarin arm vs 14.9% in the rivaroxaban arm
ARISTOTLE[49]	Warfarin (INR 2.0–3.0) vs apixaban 5 mg bid [b]	Stroke or systemic embolism, major bleeding per ISTH	1.60% In the warfarin arm vs 1.27% in the apixaban arm	3.09% In the warfarin arm vs 2.13% in the apixaban arm

ISTH definition of major bleeding: clinically overt bleeding accompanied by a decrease in the hemoglobin level of at least 2 g per dL or transfusion of at least 2 units of packed red cells, occurring at a critical site or resulting in death.
[a] The dose of rivaroxaban was reduced to 15 mg daily in patients with a creatinine clearance of 30–49 mL/min.
[b] The dose of apixaban was reduced to 2.5 mg bid in patients who had at least 2 of the following: age ≥80 years, body weight ≤60 kg, and serum creatinine ≤1.5 mg/dL.

intracranial or retroperitoneal). A meta-analysis, including RCTs conducted from 1989 through and 2011 investigating the use of VKAs and newer OACs for stroke prevention, and 31 observational studies published between 2001 and 2011 assessed the bleeding risk in patients taking various OACs. The overall median incidence of major bleeding in the included RCTs was 2.1 per 100 patient-years (range 0.9–3.4 per 100 patent-years and interquartile range 1.5–3.1 per 100 patient-years). The incidence of major bleeding in the observational studies was also similar to that in the RCTs (median 2.0 per 100 patient-years; range 0.2–7.6 per 100 patient-years; and interquartile range 1.5–3.8 per 100 patient-years).[57]

The definition of major bleeding varied more across the observational studies; some studies focused predominantly on gastrointestinal bleeding and other studies emphasized bleeding from other anatomic sites.[58–60] In routine clinical practice, a major factor that also contributes to an increased risk of bleeding is the concurrent use of medications that have a tendency to interact with VKAs.[61]

Bleeding Risk with Antiplatelet Regimen and Dual Antiplatelet Therapy

In the SPAF-I trial, the incidence of major bleeding in the ASA (325 mg/d) was 1.4% per year compared with 1.6% per year in the placebo arm.[39]

In the ACTIVE W trial, the rate of major bleeding was similar in the aspirin + clopidogrel arm compared with the OAC arm (2.42% per year vs 2.21% per year, respectively; relative risk [RR] 1.10; 95% CI, 0.83–1.45; $P = .53$); however, the incidence of minor bleeds (13.58% per year vs 11.45% per year; RR 1.23; 95% CI, 1.09–1.39; $P = .0009$) and overall bleeding (15.41% per year vs 13.21% per year; RR 1.21; 95% CI, 1.08–1.35; $P = .01$) was higher with the combination of antiplatelet agents.[40,41] In the AFASAK 2 trial, the incidence of major bleeding was 0.3% and 1.4% in the warfarin + aspirin and aspirin arms, respectively,[62] the results of these RCTs suggest that the overall benefit of ASA for the prevention of stroke is limited and is even further offset by the increased risk of bleeding.

A study by Hansen and colleagues[63] based on a nationwide registry on AF patients concluded that the overall incidence of bleeding events was the highest for dual antiplatelet therapy and warfarin therapy; using warfarin monotherapy as a reference, the HR (95% CI) for the overall bleeding events was 0.93 (0.88–0.98) for aspirin, 1.06 (0.87–1.29) for clopidogrel, 1.66 (1.34–2.04) for aspirin-clopidogrel, 1.83 (1.72–1.96) for warfarin-aspirin, 3.08 (2.32–3.91) for warfarin-clopidogrel, and 3.70 (2.89–4.76) for warfarin-aspirin-clopidogrel.

As expected, the risk of bleeding complications has increased in the setting of combination of antiplatelet agents and OACs; this is particularly relevant in the routine clinical practice where it is likely for patients to be on multiple agents, leading to an increased risk of bleeding complications.[64] In a subsequent analysis of the RE-LY trial, the use of antiplatelet agents in addition to dabigatran (110 mg), dabigatran (150 mg), and dose-adjusted warfarin was found associated with an increased risk of bleeding (overall HR 2.01; 95% CI, 1.79–2.25); also, the risk of bleeding was greater with the use of dual antiplatelet agents (HR 2.31; 95% CI, 1.79–2.98) compared with a single antiplatelet agent (HR 1.60; 95% CI, 1.42–1.82). The addition of either single or dual antiplatelet agent was not observed to have any additional beneficial effect toward the prevention of stroke and systemic embolism in the dabigatran arm compared with warfarin.[65]

Bleeding Risk with Warfarin and Newer OACs

In the SPAF-I, the rate of major bleeding was 1.2% per year in the warfarin arm.[39] The cumulative risk of major bleeding events after 3 years of treatment was 24.7% in patients receiving minidose warfarin (1.25 mg/d) and 41.1% in the adjusted-dose warfarin (to maintain an INR of 2.0–3.0) in the AFASAK 2 trial.[42,62] Similar results of increased bleeding events were reported in the ACTIVE W trial—2.02% per year in the warfarin arm. An important observation based on the results of the ACTIVE W trial is that the patients who were taking warfarin therapy at the time of enrollment in the clinical trial had a lower incidence of major bleeding (2.02%) compared with patients who were naïve to warfarin therapy at the time of enrollment in the clinical trial (2.92%); this could be due to a better drug compliance and lesser variations in the INR of the patients with previous exposure to warfarin therapy.[40] The incidence of major bleeding events during warfarin therapy in various RCTs is summarized in **Table 2**.

In the RE-LY trial, the annual incidence of major bleeding in the warfarin arm was 3.36% compared with 2.71% in the 110-mg dabigatran arm ($P = .003$); the rate of hemorrhagic stroke was also higher in the warfarin arm (0.38% per year vs 0.12% per year in the 110-mg dabigatran arm and 0.10% per year in the 150-mg dabigatran arm; $P = .001$). The incidence of gastrointestinal bleeding was significantly higher in the dabigatran 150-mg arm (1.51% per year vs 1.02% per year in the warfarin arm; $P<.001$).[47]

In the ROCKET-AF trial, the incidence of major or clinically relevant nonmajor bleeding was similar in both rivaroxaban and warfarin arms (14.9% per year vs 14.5%, respectively; HR 1.03; 95% CI, 0.96–1.11; P = .44); the use of rivaroxaban was associated with significant reduction in intracranial hemorrhages (0.5% vs 0.7%, P = .02); in contrast, the incidence of gastrointestinal bleeding was significantly greater in the rivaroxaban arm (3.2% vs 2.2%, P<.001).[48] The finding of a significantly increased incidence of major bleeding in the warfarin arm (3.09% per year) compared with 2.13% per year in the apixaban arm (HR 0.69; 95% CI, 0.60–0.80; P<.001) in the ARISTOTLE trial was consistent with the finding of the RE-LY and ROCKET-AF trials.[49] The comparison of various bleeding events between the warfarin arm and newer OACs is summarized in **Table 3**.

Bleeding Risk–Prediction Schemes

In routine clinical practice, it becomes particularly challenging to accurately estimate a patient's risk of bleeding due to presence of common risk factors for bleeding and thromboembolism and transient nature of some risk factors (concurrent use of medications, transient illness, and an anticipated invasive procedure); also, physician-perceived bleeding risk of a patient may overestimate the risk of bleeding, which is an important contributor toward suboptimal use of OACs in the AF patient population.[66,67]

To facilitate bleeding risk assessment process, various bleeding prediction schemes have been devised. The HEMORR$_2$HAGES score was devised from a Medicare database consisting of AF patients on OACs accounting for hospitalizations due to bleeding episodes.[68] The score awards 2 points for a prior bleed and 1 point for each of the other risk factors (**Box 2**).

To improve the user-friendliness of this score, the HAS-BLED score (**Box 3**) was devised based on the risk factors of bleeding identified from a cohort of 3978 patients in the Euro Heart Survey on AF and other established risk factors from systematic reviews and multivariate analyses (**Table 4**).[69–71]

The HAS-BLED score demonstrated a good predictive accuracy in the overall Euro Heart survey cohort (C statistic 0.72) and performed particularly well in patients where antiplatelet therapy was used alone (C statistic 0.91) or who had no antithrombotic therapy at all (C statistic 0.85). This score also has key advantages over the HEMORR$_2$HAGES score: first, the shorter acronym makes it easier for physicians to memorize, thereby increasing the user-friendliness and

---

Box 2
The HEMORR$_2$HAGES bleeding risk score

Hepatic or renal disease	1 Point
Ethanol abuse	1 Point
Malignancy	1 Point
Older age >75 years	1 Point
Reduced platelet count or function	1 Point
Rebleeding risk	2 Points
Hypertension (uncontrolled)	1 Point
Anemia	1 Point
Genetic factors	1 Point
Excessive fall risk	1 Point
Stroke	1 Point

Data from Gage BF, Yan Y, Milligan PE, et al. Clinical classification schemes for predicting hemorrhage: results from the National Registry of Atrial Fibrillation (NRAF). Am Heart J 2006;151:715.

Box 3
The HAS-BLED bleeding risk score

Hypertension	1 Point
Abnormal renal and liver function	1 Point each
Stroke	1 Point
Bleeding	1 Point
Labile INRs	1 Point
Elderly	1 Point
Drugs or alcohol	1 Point each

Hypertension defined as systolic blood pressure >160 mm Hg.

Abnormal renal function defined as the presence of chronic dialysis or renal transplantation or serum creatinine >200 μmol/L.

Abnormal liver function defined as chronic hepatic disease (eg, cirrhosis) and biochemical evidence of significant hepatic derangement (eg, bilirubin >2× upper limit of the normal) in association with aspartate transaminase/alanine transaminase/alkaline phosphatase >3× upper limit of the normal.

Bleeding refers to previous bleeding history or predisposition to bleeding or predisposition to bleeding (bleeding diathesis or anemia).

Labile INR: unstable/high INRs or poor time in therapeutic range (eg, <60%).

Drugs/alcohol use refers to concomitant use of drugs, such as antiplatelet agents, nonsteroidal antiinflammatory drugs and alcohol consumption of >8 units alcohol every week.

Data from Pisters R, Lane DA, Nieuwlaat R, et al. A novel user-friendly score (HAS-BLED) to assess 1-year risk of major bleeding in patients with atrial fibrillation: the Euro Heart Survey. Chest 2010;138:1095.

Table 4
The risk of major bleeding in patients with atrial fibrillation enrolled in the Euro Heart Survey

HAS-BLED Score	Bleeds per 100 Patient-Years
0	1.13
1	1.02
2	1.88
3	3.74
4	8.70

Data from Pisters R, Lane DA, Nieuwlaat R, et al. A novel user-friendly score (HAS-BLED) to assess 1-year risk of major bleeding in patients with atrial fibrillation: the Euro Heart Survey. Chest 2010;138:1097.

subsequent clinical application; and second, in contrast to the risk factors incorporated into the HEMORR$_2$HAGES score, which require laboratory parameters and genetic testing, various risk factors of the HAS-BLED score are readily available from the medical history or routinely tested in AF patients. In the overall AF population, the predictive accuracy of the HAS-BLED score has been found comparable to the HEMORR$_2$HAGES score (C statistic 0.72 vs 0.66, respectively).

In 2011, the Anticoagulation and Risk Factors in Atrial Fibrillation (ATRIA) study group described a new bleeding risk scheme for AF, as shown in **Box 4**.[72] Although the ATRIA score was simple to use, it had several limitations: first, the score was derived from a cohort exclusively consisting of anticoagulated AF patients; second, the rate of bleeding in a warfarin-experienced cohort could have been underestimated compared with warfarin-naïve patients; and third, the study did not account for data about the intensity of

Box 4
The ATRIA bleeding risk score

Anemia	3 Points
Severe renal disease (estimated GFR <30 mL/min)	3 Points
Age ≥75 years	2 Points
Prior hemorrhage	1 Point
Hypertension	1 Point

Anemia was defined according to the *International Classification of Diseases, Ninth Revision, Clinical Modification* codes.
Abbreviation: GFR, glomerular filtration rate.
Data from Fang MC, Go AS, Chang Y, et al. A new risk scheme to predict warfarin-associated hemorrhage: the ATRIA (Anticoagulation and Risk Factors in Atrial Fibrillation) Study. J Am Coll Cardiol 2011;58:399.

anticoagulation effect (ie, quality of INR control) and concomitant use of medications, such as antiplatelet and nonsteroidal antiinflammatory drugs, which are important risk factors for bleeding.[73]

The predictive value of the HAS-BLED and ATRIA scores for bleeding risk was compared in a prospective study based on a cohort of 937 AF patients from an outpatient anticoagulation clinic; over a median follow-up period of 952 days, the HAS-BLED score was found superior to the ATRIA score for prediction of bleeding risk (C statistic 0.68 vs 0.59; $P = .035$)[74]; however, in another prospective validation study on 515 patients on oral anticoagulation followed over a period of 12 months, none of the 7 bleeding risk–prediction scores was demonstrated superior than another or physician subjective risk assessment of bleeding (**Table 5**).[75]

There are considerations that should be kept in mind while using the HAS-BLED score in clinical practice: first, in patients who have a high HAS-BLED score (≥3), the risk of stroke is still high and merely a high HAS-BLED score should not be the only consideration for lack of prescription of OACs[76,77]; and, second, the dynamic nature of HAS-BLED score should also be considered based on the correctable variables (such as, in the HAS-BLED, uncontrolled blood pressure, H; labile INR, L; and concomitant use of antiplatelet drugs, D) incorporated in the score. These variables can be addressed to reduce the bleeding risk and the process of bleeding and, therefore, stroke risk assessment should be repeated at regular intervals in clinical practice. Despite the bleeding risk in patients with high HAS-BLED scores, the net clinical benefit of preventing ischemic stroke is greater than the bleeding risk and favors the use of OACs in these patients given their increased risk of stroke.[78]

In a recently published study based on 10,098 AF patients from the Outcomes Registry for Better Informed Treatment of Atrial Fibrillation (ORBIT-AF), the use of OACs was analyzed according to the CHADS$_2$ and ATRIA scores. The results of this study suggested that the overall decision to anticoagulate AF patients was predominantly driven by stroke risk rather than bleeding risk; the increase in OAC use, moving from low to high stroke risk strata, was greater than the decrease in OACs, moving from low to high bleeding risk; the rates of OACs decreased from 76.9 % to 73.4 % among all patients with low versus high ATRIA scores; in contrast, the rates of OACs increased from 66.1% to 80.0% in patients with low versus high CHADS$_2$ scores; furthermore, the rates of OACs increased more moving from low to high CHADS$_2$ scores among

Table 5
Relative comparison of various bleeding risk–prediction schemes in patients with atrial fibrillation

Bleeding Score	Major Bleeding Definition	C Statistic and 95% CI of Score Performance Based on a Prospective Validation Study	Categories According to Risk
HEMORR$_2$HAGES[68]	Any hospitalization for hemorrhage determined by Medicare claims	0.58 (0.50–0.67)	Low: 0–1 Intermediate: 2–3 High: ≥4
HAS-BLED[69]	Any bleeding requiring hospitalization or causing a decrease in hemoglobin level >20 g/L or requiring blood transfusion that was not a hemorrhagic stroke	0.57 (0.49–0.65)	Low: 0 Intermediate: 1–2 High: ≥3
ATRIA[72]	Fatal bleeding, requiring transfusion ≥2 units of blood or into a critical anatomic site	0.61 (0.52–0.70)	Low: 0–3 Intermediate: 4 High: 5–10

Data from Donzé N, Rodondi N, Waeber G, et al. Scores to predict major bleeding risk during oral anticoagulation therapy: a prospective validation study. Am J Med 2012;125:1097–8.

Table 6
Rates of anticoagulation according to stroke and bleeding risk in the ORBIT-AF study

ATRIA Score[a]	CHADS$_2$ Score[a] Low (0–1), n/N (%)	CHADS$_2$ Score High (≥2), n/N (%)	Total n/N (%)
Low (0–3)	1633/2548 (66.4)	4011/4884 (82.1)	5644/7342 (76.9)
High (≥4)	261/409 (63.8)	1656/2202 (75.2)	1917/2611 (73.4)
Total	1894/2867 (66.1)	5667/7086 (80.0)	7561/9953 (76.0)

[a] The components of ATRIA and CHADS$_2$ scores are described in **Box 4** and **Box 3**, respectively.
    From Cullen MW, Kim S, Piccini JP Sr, et al, on behalf of the ORBIT-AF Investigators. Risks and benefits of anticoagulation in atrial fibrillation: Insights from the Outcomes Registry for Better Informed Treatment of Atrial Fibrillation (ORBIT-AF) Registry. Circ Cardiovasc Qual Outcomes 2013;6(4):465; with permission.

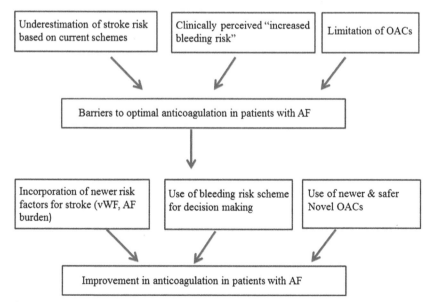

Fig. 2. Role of various factors leading to suboptimal anticoagulation for thromboprophylaxis in patients with nonvalvular AF.

patients with low bleeding risk compared with patients with higher bleeding risk (**Table 6**).[79]

The results of this study also highlight the phenomenon that the patients who are at highest stroke risk are still less likely to receive OACs. Although it seems intuitive for physicians to adopt a conservative approach of do no harm while prescribing OACs to AF patients who are at high bleeding risk, currently available data suggest that the net benefit of OAC use is greater than its risk through reduction in stroke risk (**Fig. 2**).[78,80,81]

SUMMARY

In routine clinical practice, physicians are faced with the challenge of making decisions about initiation and management of OAC therapy for stroke prevention in patients with AF. Currently available data strongly favor the use of OACs for prevention of stroke in patients with AF except for those who are at truly low risk (patients with a CHA_2DS_2-VASc score of 0). Patients who are at an increased bleeding risk (patients with a high HAS-BLED score >3) are also at increased risk of stroke,

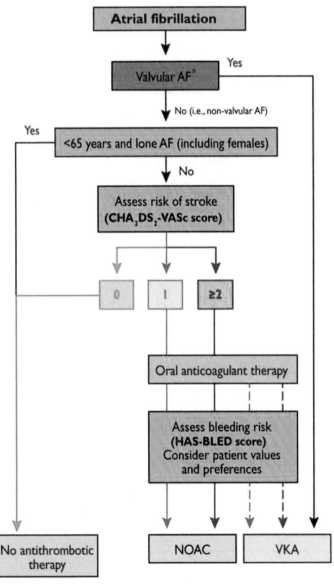

Fig. 3. Choice of anticoagulant. Initial focus on identification of truly low risk (ie, age <65) years and lone AF (irrespective of gender) or CHA_2DS_2-VASc score = 0. Female patients who are aged less than 65 years and have lone AF (but still have CHA_2DS_2-VASc score = 1 by virtue of their gender) are at low risk and no antithrombotic therapy should be considered. Solid line, best option; dashed line, alternative option. CHA_2DS_2-VASc, see text; HAS-BLED, see text; NOAC, novel OAC. (*From* Camm AJ, Lip GY, De Catarina R, et al. 2012 Focused update of the ESC guidelines for the management of atrial fibrillation: an update of the 2010 ESC guidelines for the management of atrial fibrillation. Europace 2012;14:1395; with permission.)

Colour: CHA_2DS_2-VASc; green = 0, blue = 1, red = 2.

[a] Includes rheumatic valvular disease and prosthetic valves.

and the benefit of OAC therapy in these patients is greater than the risk of bleeding. A strategy that combines clinical decision making based on evaluation of a patient's risks of stroke and bleeding based on risk-prediction schemes and patient preferences and compliance should be used for the selection of appropriate stroke prophylaxis for patients with AF (**Fig. 3**).[81] The choice of anticoagulant therapy for stroke prophylaxis in patients with AF is best individualized and should consider a patient's inherent stroke risk and the accurate estimate of absolute benefits as well as bleeding risk, access to high-quality anticoagulation monitoring, and patient preferences.

REFERENCES

1. Chugh SS, Blackshear JL, Shen WK, et al. Epidemiology and natural history of atrial fibrillation: clinical implications. J Am Coll Cardiol 2001;37:371–8.

2. Krahn AD, Manfreda J, Tate RB, et al. The natural history of atrial fibrillation: incidence, risk factors and prognosis in the Manitoba Follow-Up Study. Am J Med 1995;98:476–84.

3. Wolf PA, Abbott RD, Kannel WB. Atrial fibrillation as an independent risk factor for stroke: the Framingham Study. Stroke 1991;22:983–8.

4. Hart RG, Pearce LA, Aguilar MI. Meta-analysis: Antithrombotic therapy to prevent stroke in patients who have nonvalvular atrial fibrillation. Ann Intern Med 2007;146:857–67.

5. Poli D, Antonucci E, Marcucci R, et al. Risk of bleeding in very old atrial fibrillation patients on warfarin: relationship with ageing and CHADS2 score. Thromb Res 2007;121:347–52.

6. Hughes M, Lip GY. Risk factors for anticoagulation-related bleeding complications in patients with atrial fibrillation: a systematic review. QJM 2007; 100:599–607.

7. Lip GY, Andreotti F, Fauchier L, et al. Bleeding risk assessment and management in atrial fibrillation patients: a position document from the European Heart Rhythm Association, endorsed by the European Society of Cardiology working group on Thrombosis. Europace 2011;13:723–46.

8. Lopes LC, Spencer PA, Neumann I, et al. Bleeding risk in atrial fibrillation patients taking vitamin K antagonists: systematic review and meta-analysis. Clin Pharmacol Ther 2013;94(3):367–75.

9. Topcuoglu MA, Haydari D, Oztruk S, et al. Plasma levels of coagulation and fibrinolysis markers in acute ischemic stroke patients with lone atrial fibrillation. Neurol Sci 2000;21:235–40.

10. Fu R, Wu S, Wu P, et al. A study of blood soluble P-selectin, fibrinogen, and vonWillebrand factor levels in idiopathic and lone atrial fibrillation. Europace 2011;13:31–6.

11. Matsumoto M, Sakaguchi M, Okazaki S, et al. Relationship between plasma (D)- dimer level and cerebral infarction volume in patients with nonvalvular atrial fibrillation. Cerebrovasc Dis 2013;35:64–72.

12. Kumagai K, Fukunami M, Ohmori M, et al. Increased intracardiovascular clotting in patients with chronic atrial fibrillation. J Am Coll Cardiol 1990;16:377–80.

13. Scridon A, Girerd N, Rugeri L, et al. Progressive endothelial damage revealed by multilevel von Willebrand factor plasma concentrations in atrial fibrillation patients. Europace 2013;15(11):1562–6.

14. Hayashi M, Takeshita K, Inden Y, et al. Platelet activation and induction of tissue factor in acute and chronic atrial fibrillation: involvement of mononuclear cell-platelet interaction. Thromb Res 2011; 128:e113–8.

15. Cotter PE, Martin PJ, Ring L, et al. Incidence of atrial fibrillation detected by implantable loop recorders in unexplained stroke. Neurology 2013; 80:1546–50.

16. Sinha AM, Diener HC, Morillo CA, et al. Cryptogenic stroke and underlying Atrial Fibrillation (CRYSTAL AF): design and rationale. Am Heart J 2010;160:36–41.

17. Stroke Risk in Atrial Fibrillation Working Group. Independent predictors of stroke in patients with atrial fibrillation: a systematic review. Neurology 2007;69:546–54.

18. Hughes M, Lip GY. Stroke and thromboembolism in atrial fibrillation: a systematic review of the stroke risk factors, risk stratification schema and cost effectiveness data. Thromb Haemost 2008;99: 295–304.

19. Karthikeyan G, Eikelbloom JW. The CHADS2 score for stroke risk stratification in atrial fibrillation- friend or foe? Thromb Haemost 2010;104:657–63.

20. Lip GY, Nieuwlaat R, Pisters R, et al. Refining clinical risk stratification for predicting stroke and thromboembolism in atrial fibrillation using a novel risk factor-based approach: the euro heart survey on atrial fibrillation. Chest 2010;137:263–72.

21. Rasmussen LH, Larsen TB, Due KM, et al. Impact of vascular disease in predicting stroke and death in patients with atrial fibrillation: the Danish Diet, Cancer and Health cohort study. J Thromb Haemost 2011;9:1301–7.

22. Olesen JB, Fauchier L, Lane DA, et al. Risk factors for stroke and thromboembolism in relation to age among patients with atrial fibrillation: the Loire Valley Atrial fibrillation Project. Chest 2012; 141:147–53.

23. European Heart Rhythm Association, European Association for Cardio-Thoracic Surgery, Camm AJ, Kirchhof P, Lip GY, et al. Guidelines for the management of atrial fibrillation: the Task force for the management of atrial fibrillation of

the European Society of Cardiology. Eur Heart J 2010;31:2369–429.

24. Lip GY, Halperin JL. Improving risk stratification in atrial fibrillation. Am J Med 2010;123:484–8.

25. Sadler JE. Biochemistry and genetics of von Willebrand factor. Annu Rev Biochem 1998;67:395–424.

26. Kanaji S, Fahs SA, Shi Q, et al. Contribution of platelet vs. endothelial VWF to platelet adhesion and hemostasis. J Thromb Haemost 2012;10:1646–52.

27. Blann A. von Willebrand factor and the endothelium in vascular disease. Br J Biomed Sci 1993;50:125–34.

28. Lip GY, Lowe GD, Rumley A, et al. Increased markers of thrombogenesis in chronic atrial fibrillation: effects of warfarin treatment. Br Heart J 1995;73:527–33.

29. Conway DS, Pearce LA, Chin BS, et al. Plasma von Willebrand factor and soluble P-Selectin as indices of endothelial damage and platelet activation in 1321 patients with nonvalvular atrial fibrillation: relationship to stroke risk factors. Circulation 2002;106:1962–7.

30. Wieberdink RG, van Schie MC, Koudstaal PJ, et al. High von Willebrand factor levels increases the risk of stroke: the Rotterdam study. Stroke 2010;41:2151–6.

31. Adjusted-dose warfarin versus low-intensity, fixed-dose warfarin plus aspirin for high-risk patients with atrial fibrillation: Stroke Prevention in Atrial Fibrillation III randomised clinical trial. Lancet 1996;348:633–8.

32. Atrial Fibrillation Investigators. Risk factors for stroke and efficiency of antithrombotic therapy in atrial fibrillation: analysis of pooled data from five randomised trials. Arch Intern Med 1994;154:1449–57.

33. Lip GY, Lane D, Van Walraven C, et al. Additive role of plasma von Willebrand factor levels to clinical factors for risk stratification of patients with atrial fibrillation. Stroke 2006;37:2294–300.

34. Mukamal KJ, Tolstrup JS, Friberg J, et al. Fibrinogen and albumin levels and risk of atrial fibrillation in men and women (the Copenhagen City Heart Study). Am J Cardiol 2006;98:75–81.

35. Sohara H, Amitani S, Kurose M, et al. Atrial fibrillation activates platelets and coagulation in a time-dependent manner: a study in patients with paroxysmal atrial fibrillation. J Am Coll Cardiol 1997;29:106–12.

36. Flaker GC, Belew K, Beckman K, et al, AFFIRM Investigators. Asymptomatic atrial fibrillation: demographic features and prognostic information from the Atrial Fibrillation Follow-up Investigation of Rhythm Management (AFFIRM) study. Am Heart J 2005;149:657–63.

37. Glotzer TV, Hellkamp AS, Zimmerman J, et al, MOST Investigators. Atrial high rate episodes detected by pacemaker diagnostics predict death and stroke: report of the Atrial Diagnostics Ancillary Study of the Mode Selection Trial (MOST). Circulation 2003;107:1614–9.

38. Petersen P, Boysen G, Godtfredsen J, et al. Placebo-controlled, randomised trial of warfarin and aspirin for prevention of thromboembolic complications in chronic atrial fibrillation. The Copenhagen AFASAK study. Lancet 1989;1:175–9.

39. Stroke Prevention in Atrial Fibrillation Investigators. Stroke prevention in atrial fibrillation study. Final results. Circulation 1991;84:527–39.

40. ACTIVE Writing Group of the ACTIVE Investigators, Connolly S, Pogue J, Hart R, et al. Clopidogrel plus aspirin versus oral anticoagulation for atrial fibrillation in the Atrial Fibrillation Clopidogrel Trial with Irbesartan for prevention of Vascular Events (ACTIVE W): a randomised controlled trial. Lancet 2006;367:1903–12.

41. ACTIVE Investigators, Connolly S, Pogue J, Hart R, et al. Effect of clopidogrel added to aspirin in patients with atrial fibrillation. N Engl J Med 2009;360:2066–78.

42. Gullov AL, Koefoed BG, Petersen P, et al. Fixed minidose warfarin and aspirin alone and in combination vs. adjusted-dose warfarin for stroke prevention in atrial fibrillation: second Copenhagen Atrial Fibrillation, Aspirin, and Anticoagulation Study. Arch Intern Med 1998;158:1513–21.

43. Chaudhury A, Lip GY. Atrial fibrillation and the hypercoagulable state: from basic science to clinical practice. Pathophysiol Haemost Thromb 2003;33:282–9.

44. Watson T, Shantsila E, Lip GY. Mechanisms of thrombogenesis in atrial fibrillation: Virchow's triad revisited. Lancet 2009;373:155–66.

45. Benbir G, Uluduz D, Ince B, et al. Atherothrombotic ischemic stroke in patients with atrial fibrillation. Clin Neurol Neurosurg 2007;109:485–90.

46. Connolly SJ, Laupacis A, Gent M, et al. Candian atrial fibrillation anticoagulation (CAFA) study. J Am Coll Cardiol 1991;18:349–55.

47. Connolly SJ, Ezekowitz MD, Yusuf S, et al, RE-LY Steering Committee and Investigators. Dabigatran versus warfarin in patients with atrial fibrillation. N Engl J Med 2009;361:1139–51.

48. Patel MR, Mahaffey KW, Garg J, et al, ROCKET AF Investigators. Rivaroxaban versus warfarin in nonvalvular atrial fibrillation. N Engl J Med 2011;365:883–91.

49. Granger CB, Alexander JH, McMurray JJ, et al, ARISTOTLE Committees and Investigators. Apixaban versus warfarin in patients with atrial fibrillation. N Engl J Med 2011;365:981–92.

50. Kirchhof P, Nabauer M, Gerth A, et al, AFNET Registry Invetigators. Impact of the type of center on management of AF patients: surprising evidence of differences in antithrombotic therapy decisions. Thromb Haemost 2011;105:1010–23.

51. Wilke T, Groth A, Mueller S, et al. Oral anticoagulation use by patients with atrial fibrillation in Germany. Adherence to guidelines causes of anticoagulation under-use and its clinical outcomes, based on claims-data of 183,448 patients. Thromb Haemost 2012;107:1053–65.

52. Hylek EM, Evans-Molina C, Shea C, et al. Major hemorrhage and tolerability of warfarin in the first year of therapy among elderly patients with atrial fibrillation. Circulation 2007;115:2689–96.

53. Fang MC, Chang Y, Hylek EM, et al. Advanced age, anticoagulation intensity, and risk of intracranial hemorrhage among patients taking warfarin for atrial fibrillation. Ann Intern Med 2004;141:745–52.

54. Rosand J, Hylek EM, O'Donnell HC, et al. Warfarin-associated hemorrhage and cerebral amyloid angiopathy: a genetic and pathologic study. Neurology 2000;55:947–51.

55. Smith EE, Rosand J, Knudsen KA, et al. Leukoaraiosis is associated with warfarin-related hemorrhage following ischemic stroke. Neurology 2002;59:193–7.

56. Schulman S, Kearon C, Subcommittee on Control of Anticoagulation of the Scientific and Standardization Committee of the International Society on Thrombosis and Haemostasis. Definition of major bleeding in clinical investigations of antihemostatic medicinal products in non-surgical patients. J Thromb Haemost 2005;3:692–4.

57. Roskell NS, Samuel M, Noack H, et al. Major bleeding in patients with atrial fibrillation receiving vitamin K antagonists: a systemic review of randomized and observational studies. Europace 2013;15:787–97.

58. Cheung CM, Tsoi TH, Huang CY. The lowest effective intensity of prophylactic anticoagulation for patients with atrial fibrillation. Cerebrovasc Dis 2005;20:114–9.

59. Ghate SR, Biskupiak JE, Ye X, et al. Hemorrhagic and thrombotic events associated with generic substitution of warfarin in patients with atrial fibrillation. Ann Pharmacother 2011;45:701–12.

60. Shireman TI, Howard PA, Kresowik TF, et al. Combined anticoagulant-antiplatelet use and major bleeding events in elderly atrial fibrillation patients. Stroke 2004;35:2362–7.

61. Vitry AI, Roughead EE, Ramsay EN, et al. Major bleeding risk associated with warfarin and co-medications in the elderly population. Pharmacoepidemiol Drug Saf 2011;20:1057–63.

62. Gullov AL, Koefoed BG, Petersen P. Bleeding during warfarin and aspirin therapy in patients with atrial fibrillation: the AFASAK 2 study. Atrial fibrillation aspirin and anticoagulation. Arch Intern Med 1999;159:1322–8.

63. Hansen ML, Sorensen R, Clausen MT, et al. Risk of bleeding with single, dual, or triple therapy with warfarin, aspirin, and clopidogrel in patients with atrial fibrillation. Arch Intern Med 2010;170:1433–41.

64. Douketis JD. Combination warfarin-ASA therapy: which patients should receive it, which patients should not, and why? Thromb Res 2011;127:513–7.

65. Dans AL, Connolly SJ, Wallentin L, et al. Concomitant use of antiplatelet therapy with dabigatran or warfarin in the randomized evaluation of long-term anticoagulation therapy (RE-LY) trial. Circulation 2013;127:634–40.

66. Beyth RJ, Antani MR, Covinsky KE, et al. Why isn't warfarin prescribed to patients with nonrheumatic atrial fibrillation? J Gen Intern Med 1996;11:721–8.

67. Monette J, Gurwitz JH, Rochon PA. Physician attitude concerning warfarin for stroke prevention in atrial fibrillation: results of a survey of long-term care practitioners. J Am Geriatr Soc 1997;45:1060–5.

68. Gage BF, Yan Y, Milligan PE, et al. Clinical classification schemes for predicting hemorrhage: results from the National Registry of Atrial Fibrillation (NRAF). Am Heart J 2006;151:713–9.

69. Pisters R, Lane DA, Nieuwlaat R, et al. A novel user-friendly score (HAS-BLED) to assess one-year risk of major bleeding in patients with atrial fibrillation: the Euro Heart Survey. Chest 2010;138:1093–100.

70. Palareti G, Cosmi B. Bleeding with anticoagulation therapy- who is at risk, and how best to identify such patients. Thromb Haemost 2009;102:268–78.

71. Tay KH, Lane DA, Lip GY. Bleeding risks with combination of oral anticoagulation plus antiplatelet therapy: is clopidogrel any safer than aspirin when combined with warfarin? Thromb Haemost 2008;100:955–7.

72. Fang MC, Go AS, Chang Y, et al. A new risk scheme to predict warfarin- associated hemorrhage: the ATRIA (Anticoagulation and Risk Factors in Atrial Fibrillation) Study. J Am Coll Cardiol 2011;58:395–401.

73. Olesen JB, Pisters R, Roldans V, et al. The ATRIA risk scheme to predict warfarin-associated hemorrhage not ready for clinical use. J Am Coll Cardiol 2012;59:194–5.

74. Roldán V, Marín F, Fernández H, et al. Predictive value of the HAS-BLED and ATRIA bleeding scores for the risk of serious bleeding in a "real-world" population with atrial fibrillation receiving anticoagulant therapy. Chest 2013;143:179–84.

75. Donzé N, Rodondi N, Waeber G, et al. Scores to predict major bleeding risk during oral

anticoagulation therapy: a prospective validation study. Am J Med 2012;125:1095–102.

76. Camm AJ, Lip GY, De Catarina R, et al. 2012 focused update of the ESC guidelines for the management of atrial fibrillation: an update of the 2010 ESC guidelines for the management of atrial fibrillation. Europace 2012;14:1385–413.

77. Stott DJ, Dewar RI, Garratt CJ, et al, Royal College of Physicians of Edinburgh. RCPE UK Consensus Conference on "Approaching the comprehensive management of atrial fibrillation: evolution or revolution?". J R Coll Physicians Edinb 2012;42(Suppl 18):3–4.

78. Olesen JB, Lip GY, Lindhardsen J, et al. Risks of thromboembolism and bleeding with thromboprophylaxis in patients with atrial fibrillation: a net clinical benefit analysis using a "real world" nationwide cohort study. Thromb Haemost 2011;106: 739–49.

79. Cullen MW, Kim S, Piccini JP Sr, et al, on behalf of the ORBIT-AF Investigators. Risks and benefits of anticoagulation in atrial fibrillation: insights from the Outcomes Registry for Better Informed Treatment of Atrial Fibrillation (ORBIT-AF) Registry. Circ Cardiovasc Qual Outcomes 2013;6(4):461–9.

80. Singer DE, Chang Y, Fang MC, et al. The net clinical benefit of warfarin anticoagulation in atrial fibrillation. Ann Intern Med 2009;151:297–305.

81. Friberg L, Rosenqvist M, Lip GY. Net clinical benefit of warfarin in patients with atrial fibrillation: a report from the Swedish atrial fibrillation cohort study. Circulation 2012;125:2298–307.

Embryology and Anatomy of the Left Atrial Appendage
Why Does Thrombus Form?

Arun Kanmanthareddy, MD, MS[a], Yeruva Madhu Reddy, MD[b],
Ajay Vallakati, MD[c], Matthew B. Earnest, MD[d], Jayant Nath, MD[a],
Ryan Ferrell, MD[a], Buddhadeb Dawn, MD[a],
Dhanunjaya Lakkireddy, MD, FHRS[e,*]

KEYWORDS

• Left atrial appendage • LAA thrombus • LAA dysfunction • LAA size and volume • Atrial fibrillation

KEY POINTS

• Thrombus formation in the left atrial appendage (LAA) is caused by the complex interplay of anatomic and histologic changes in the LAA combined with the altered procoagulant state during atrial fibrillation (AF).
• Assessment of LAA anatomy and function may be considered in addition to CHADS$_2$ (congestive heart failure, hypertension, age, diabetes, prior stroke) and CHA$_2$DS$_2$-Vasc (congestive heart failure, hypertension, age ≥75 years, diabetes mellitus, stroke, vascular disease, age 65–74 years, sex category) to estimate the risk of thromboembolism and the need for anticoagulation in AF.
• Knowledge about LAA anatomy is important when patients are being considered for LAA ligation and closure devices.

INTRODUCTION

The left atrial appendage (LAA) is a blind tubular structure arising from the left atrium (LA) and it represents the primitive LA. The critical role of LAA in the formation of thrombus in patients with atrial fibrillation (AF) is well established. In addition, it is also proposed to be an uncommon site for the initiation and maintenance of AF.[1] It is reported that approximately 57% of LA thrombi in rheumatic heart disease and 91% of thrombi in nonrheumatic AF originate from the LAA.[2] LAA being a common site of LA thrombus has been attributed to its complex anatomic, histologic, and functional characteristics. The roles of various factors involved in the thrombus formation in LAA are shown in **Fig. 1**. This article reviews the embryology, anatomy, and proposed local and systemic factors that play a role in thrombus formation in the LAA.

EMBRYOLOGY OF THE LAA

During the third week of development, a pair of endocardial tubes is formed on either side of the midline by the endocardial cells derived from the

The authors have nothing to disclose.
[a] Division of Cardiovascular Medicine, Mid-America Cardiology, University of Kansas Hospital, University of Kansas Medical Center, Kansas City, KS 66160, USA; [b] Division of Cardiovascular Medicine, University of Kansas Hospital, Kansas City, KS 66160, USA; [c] Division of Cardiology, Metro Health Medical Center, Case Western Reserve University, Cleveland, OH 44109, USA; [d] Mid-America Cardiology, University of Kansas Hospital, Kansas City, KS 66160, USA; [e] Division of Cardiology, Mid-America Cardiology, Center for Excellence in Atrial Fibrillation & Electrophysiology Research, Bloch Heart Rhythm Center, KU Cardiovascular Research Institute, University of Kansas Hospital, University of Kansas Medical Center, 3901 Rainbow Boulevard, Kansas City, KS 66160, USA
* Corresponding author.
E-mail address: dlakkireddy@kumc.edu

Intervent Cardiol Clin 3 (2014) 191–202
http://dx.doi.org/10.1016/j.iccl.2013.11.002
2211-7458/14/$ – see front matter © 2014 Elsevier Inc. All rights reserved.

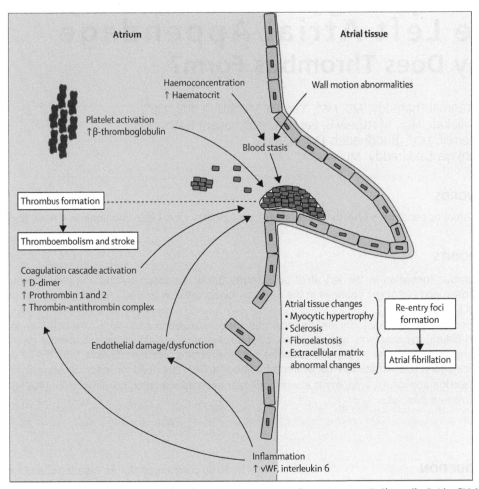

Fig. 1. Components of the Virchow triad for thrombogenesis in AF. (*From* Watson T, Shantsila E, Lip GY. Mechanisms of thrombogenesis in atrial fibrillation: Virchow's triad revisited. Lancet 2009;373(9658):156; with permission.)

splanchnopleuric mesoderm.[3] Lateral folding of the embryo results in fusion of both these tubes along with their myocardium in the midline ventrally to form the primitive heart, which is a single tubelike structure (**Fig. 2**).[3] Future structures of the heart are demarcated by constrictions on the heart tube.[4] The primitive atrium connects to the sinus venosus and lies in caudal position, whereas the bulbus cordis is cephalic and extends into the truncus arteriosus.[4] The primitive ventricle lies between these two structures.

The heart tube undergoes looping on approximately day 23 of development and the primitive atrium moves posteriorly behind the bulboventricular segment (see **Fig. 2**).[4] Until this time, the primitive atrium is outside the pericardial sac and, with further looping, it comes to lie inside the pericardial sac in a position posterosuperior to the primitive ventricle (see **Fig. 2**).[4] The primitive LA is a strong pumping structure aided by the presence of

pectinate muscles. During a process called intussusception, the right sinus bud incorporates into the primitive right atrium and the pulmonary vein (PV) bud incorporates into the primitive LA.[3] Thus the LA is formed from the fusion of PV bud and the primitive LA. The smooth wall of the LA is derived from the PVs, whereas the trabeculated primitive LA persists as the LAA (**Fig. 3**).[5]

ANATOMIC FEATURES

The LAA is a fingerlike multilobed structure that lies enclosed within the pericardium (**Fig. 4**).[6] The LAA can be grossly divided into the (1) ostium, (2) neck, and (3) the body. The LAA communicates with the LA by means of an ostium.[7] The ostial size and shape are variable. Oval shapes were most common type in 69% of the subjects in one series.[8] The neck is the narrowest part and continues into the body of the LAA.[9] The body is multilobed,

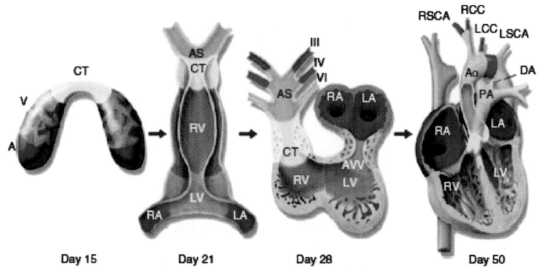

Fig. 2. Cardiac development with color coding of morphologically related regions, seen from a ventral view. Cardiogenic precursors form a crescent (left-most panel) that forms specific segments of the linear heart tube, which is patterned along the anterior-posterior axis to form the various regions and chambers of the looped and mature heart. Each cardiac chamber balloons out from the outer curvature of the looped heart tube in a segmental fashion. Neural crest cells populate the bilaterally symmetric aortic arch arteries (III, IV, and VI) and aortic sac (AS) that together contribute to specific segments of the mature aortic arch. Mesenchymal cells form the cardiac valves from the conotruncal (CT) and atrioventricular valve segments. Corresponding days of human embryonic development are indicated. A, atrium; Ao, aorta; DA, ductus arteriosus; LCC, left common carotid; LSCA, left subclavian artery; LV, left ventricle; PA, pulmonary artery; RA, right atrium; RCC, right common carotid; RSCA, right subclavian artery; RV, right ventricle; V, ventricle. (*From* Pan J, Baker KM. Retinoic acid and the heart. Vitam Horm 2007;75:259; with permission.)

with 80% of LAAs having 2 or more lobes, and these lobes extend in multiple directions.[10] LAAs have been classified into various morphologies based on their shapes on computed tomography

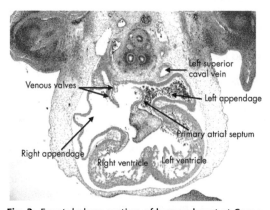

Fig. 3. Frontal plane section of human heart at Carnegie stage 16. The section shows development of the LAA from the superior aspect of the primitive LA. (*From* Moorman A, Webb S, Brown NA, et al. Development of the heart: (1) formation of the cardiac chambers and arterial trunks. Heart 2003;89(7):809; with permission.)

(CT)/magnetic resonance imaging (MRI) imaging by Wang and colleagues,[8] and Di Biase and colleagues[11] (**Table 1**). The types are (1) cactus, (2) chicken wing, (3) windsock, and (4) cauliflower (**Figs. 5–8**).[11] The chicken wing was the most common type and was present in 48% of their study patients.[11]

The epicardial surface is crenellated and lies in close proximity to the pulmonary trunk on its superior aspect and free wall of the left ventricle inferomedially.[6] The left coronary artery and great cardiac vein traverse the left atrioventricular groove under the LAA. The left coronary artery bifurcates in close proximity to the LAA into left circumflex and left anterior descending arteries. The external position of the ostium is above the atrioventricular groove.[9] The tip of the LAA is usually directed anteriorly and cephalad and it often overlaps the base of the pulmonary trunk, but it can also be directed in other directions.[9] Outside the pericardium, the left phrenic nerve along with its vascular bundle runs in close proximity to the LAA on the posterolateral aspect.[12]

The internal position of the ostium is in close proximity to the left PVs. There is a ridge between the left superior PV opening and the ostium of LAA,

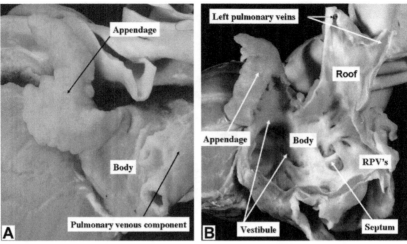

Fig. 4. The anatomy of the LA and LAA. (*A*) The tubular nature of the left appendage. (*B*) The interior of the atrium is shown having reflected the pulmonary venous component, which forms the atrial roof. RPV, right pulmonary vein. (*From* Mommersteeg MT, Christoffels VM, Anderson RH, et al. Atrial fibrillation: a developmental point of view. Heart Rhythm 2009;6(12):1819; with permission.)

which is an infolding of the left atrial wall and contains the remnant of the vein of Marshall, epicardial nerve fibers, and ganglia.[12] This ridge has been referred to as left taenia terminalis, left posterior crest, and Coumadin/warfarin ridge by various investigators.[12–14] The endocardial surface of the LAA is lined by pectinate muscles in a network of ridges and is also crenellated.[7] Pectinate muscles increase in their size with age and more than 97%

of the pectinate muscles in the LAA become greater than or equal to 1 mm in width by adult life.[10]

Histology of the LAA

The wall of the LAA comprises epicardial, myocardial, and endocardial layers. The epicardial layer overlying the atria is thicker compared with the ventricles.[6] The myocardial layers consist of muscle bundles of varied thickness and are arranged in a whorl-like fashion, and the wall of the LAA in between the pectinate muscles is thin.[9,15] Because of the varied thickness of the muscle bundles, the endocardial surface appears irregular. The myocardial structure is similar to that found in the ventricles.[16] The endocardial layer consists of a single layer of endothelial cells, which is supported by subendocardial connective tissue.

Physiologic Function

LAA cardiocytes have high concentrations of atrial natriuretic peptide, but these are less than those in the right atrial appendage.[17] Because of its unique geometric shape, it is considered to act like a pressure gauge.[18] It has been postulated that atrial natriuretic peptide is released in response to stretch of the LAA wall and causes diuresis and thus plays a physiologic role in volume overload states.[18]

PATHOLOGIC CHANGES IN THE LAA IN AF

The LAA undergoes remodeling during AF and, in chronic AF, the LAA size increases and this

Table 1	
Classification of LAA based on morphology	
Morphologic Type	**Description**
Cactus	Predominant central lobe with secondary lobes extending in superior and inferior directions
Chicken wing	The LAA folds back on itself at some distance from the perceived left atrial ostium
Windsock	Has 1 dominant lobe of sufficient structure and may have secondary or tertiary lobes arising from the primary lobe
Cauliflower	Has limited length with irregular internal characteristics

From Wang Y, Di Biase L, Horton RP, et al. Left atrial appendage studied by computed tomography to help planning for appendage closure device placement. J Cardiovasc Electrophysiol 2010;21(9):973–82; with permission.

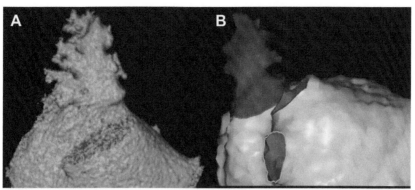

Fig. 5. CT (*A*) and MRI (*B*) scans of cactus LAA morphology. Cactus LAA morphology presents a dominant central lobe with secondary lobes extending from the central lobe in both superior and inferior directions. (*From* Di Biase L, Santangeli P, Anselmino M, et al. Does the left atrial appendage morphology correlate with the risk of stroke in patients with atrial fibrillation? Results from a multicenter study. J Am Coll Cardiol 2012;60(6):533; with permission.)

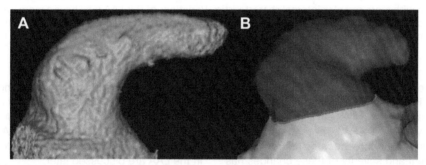

Fig. 6. CT (*A*) and MRI (*B*) scans of chicken wing LAA morphology. Chicken wing LAA morphology presents an obvious bend in the proximal or middle part of the dominant lobe, or folding back of the LAA anatomy on itself at some distance from the perceived LAA orifice. (*From* Di Biase L, Santangeli P, Anselmino M, et al. Does the left atrial appendage morphology correlate with the risk of stroke in patients with atrial fibrillation? Results from a multicenter study. J Am Coll Cardiol 2012;60(6):533; with permission.)

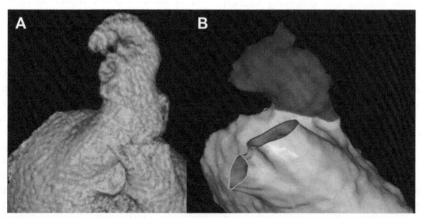

Fig. 7. CT (*A*) and MRI (*B*) scans of windsock LAA morphology. Windsock LAA morphology presents 1 dominant lobe of sufficient length as the primary structure. Variations of this LAA type arise with the location and number of secondary or even tertiary lobes. (*From* Di Biase L, Santangeli P, Anselmino M, et al. Does the left atrial appendage morphology correlate with the risk of stroke in patients with atrial fibrillation? Results from a multicenter study. J Am Coll Cardiol 2012;60(6):534; with permission.)

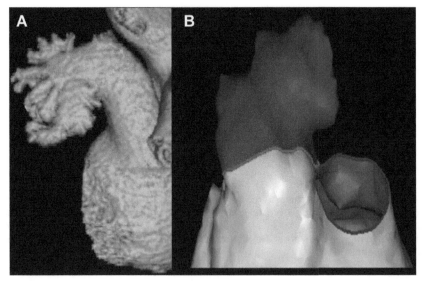

Fig. 8. CT (*A*) and MRI (*B*) scans of cauliflower LAA morphology. Cauliflower LAA morphology presents limited overall length with more complex internal characteristics. Variations of this LAA type have a more irregular shape of the LAA ostium (oval vs round). (*From* Di Biase L, Santangeli P, Anselmino M, et al. Does the left atrial appendage morphology correlate with the risk of stroke in patients with atrial fibrillation? Results from a multicenter study. J Am Coll Cardiol 2012;60(6):534; with permission.)

increase is directly proportional to the duration of AF.[19] There is hypertrophy and necrosis of the cardiomyocytes of the atria; there is also infiltration by inflammatory cells in AF.[20] These pathophysiologic changes result in endocardial fibroelastosis and the extent and severity of these changes has been found to be directly proportional to the LAA volume (**Fig. 9**).[21] Altered collagen deposition and impaired metalloproteinase activity results in encasement of the pectinate muscles by collagen.[21,22] These fibroelastotic changes depress the LAA function, which is reflected as a decrease in flow velocity and emptying fraction of the LAA.[23,24]

PREDICTORS OF THROMBOEMBOLISM

Endothelial changes and LAA dysfunction caused by fibroelastotic changes coupled with altered physiology of procoagulants and anticoagulants (local and systemic) are the three components of the Virchow triad for clot formation in the LAA. Stroke risk scoring systems such as $CHADS_2$ (congestive heart failure, hypertension, age, diabetes, prior stroke) and CHA_2DS_2-Vasc (congestive heart failure, hypertension, age $\geq$75 years, diabetes mellitus, stroke, vascular disease, age 65–74 years, sex category) are commonly used tools in clinical practice for estimating the risk of thromboembolism in AF.[25,26] These scoring systems use comorbid risk factors to assess this risk. The mechanism by which these comorbidities

contribute to thrombus formation is thought to be multifactorial. Although most of the clots in AF are found in the LAA, local factors such as size, morphology, and function of the LAA are less well studied. The factors that affect clot formation in the LAA are discussed later.

Local Factors

LAA shape and size

The non–chicken wing LAA morphology was associated with 3 times higher risk of stroke.[11] This risk is at least 6 times higher compared with the chicken wing type of LAA even in patients with a $CHADS_2$ score between 0 and 1.[11] Increase in chamber dimensions and volume of the LAA have been associated with higher stroke risk.[27] LAA volume greater than 34 cm^3 was associated with a significant increase in the risk of stroke and thromboembolism.[28] Another recent study suggests that a 10-cm^3 increase in the volume of LAA has a greater risk of stroke than a single point increase in the $CHADS_2$ score.[29] It can be hypothesized that wide chambers of the LAA probably have less turbulence and lower flow velocities, resulting in higher stasis in these cases. Recent studies have also noted that smaller ostial size increases stroke risk, possibly because of poor blood flow from the LA into the LAA resulting in stasis.[30,31] Length of the LAA was also a determinant of thromboembolism, with shorter length conferring a greater risk.[30,31]

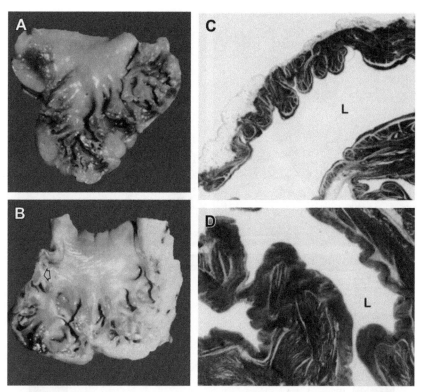

Fig. 9. Gross photograph of coronally bisected left atrial appendages in a patient in sinus rhythm (*A*) and another patient in chronic atrial fibrillation (*B*). Marked endocardial fibroelastosis is seen in the patient with atrial fibrillation (*B*) as manifested by a glistening, relatively smooth surface, encasement of pectinate muscles (*arrowhead*) and reduced relative volume of the trabeculations. Photomicrographs of histologic sections of left atrial appendage in a patient in sinus rhythm (*C*) and in another patient in chronic atrial fibrillation (*D*). Marked fibrous thickening of the endocardium is seen in the patient with atrial fibrillation with encasement of the pectinate muscles. Masson's trichrome stain. Both specimens scanned without magnification and enlarged equally at ×120. L, lumen. (*Reprinted from* Shirani J, Alaeddini J. Structural remodeling of the left atrial appendage in patients with chronic non-valvular atrial fibrillation: implications for thrombus formation, systemic embolism, and assessment by transesophageal echocardiography. Cardiovasc Pathol 2000;9(2):98; with permission from Elsevier.)

LAA dysfunction

Enlarged chamber size and fibrotic changes depress the contractile function of the LAA and cause stasis of blood.[23,32] Structural fibrotic changes in the LAA can be detected on MRI and atrial fibrosis greater than 20% had a higher likelihood of LAA thrombus.[33] LAA dysfunction can be measured indirectly by measuring its emptying fraction, peak systolic strain, and flow velocity. LAA peak systolic strain less than 21% and emptying fraction less than 21% were independent predictors of LAA thrombus and spontaneous echo contrast (SEC) (**Fig. 10**).[24,34] Antegrade flow velocity less than 20 cm/s is also associated with dense SEC and subsequent thromboembolic events.[23] The LAA velocities were higher in chicken wing–type LAA, and this may explain the lower incidence of thrombi in this type.[35] A composite scoring system to assess LAA dysfunction using left atrial volume index, left atrial ejection fraction, and LAA wall velocity has recently been proposed by Sato and colleagues.[36] Scores of greater than 2 on this scoring system were an independent predictor of thrombus formation in the LAA.

LAA function has been shown to improve following catheter ablation of AF and reverse remodeling of the LAA was noted in patients who continued to be in sinus rhythm.[37,38] This improvement in LAA function was followed by decreased SEC.[37] LAA flow velocity also depends on the rhythm. Sinus rhythm was associated with the highest flow velocities, followed by paroxysmal AF, and in chronic AF the flow velocities were significantly lower.[39] Thus, rhythm, in addition to the pathophysiologic changes in the LAA, may play a role in thrombus formation.

Role of left ventricular dysfunction in thrombus formation

A few studies have proposed that left ventricular (LV) dysfunction results in additional decrease in LAA emptying velocity.[40,41] Further, LAA thrombus

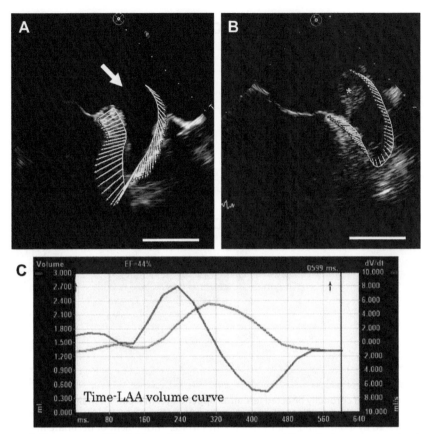

Fig. 10. Representative images of the LAA, and time-volume curve and time-strain curves constructed by velocity vector imaging in patients with AF. (*A*) LAA of a patient without thrombus (*white arrow*). (*B*) LAA of a patient with thrombus. (*C*) Time-volume curve is shown as an orange line. Time-dV/dt (rate of volume change) curve is shown as a blue line. * Thrombus. (*From* Ono K, Iwama M, Kawasaki M, et al. Motion of left atrial appendage as a determinant of thrombus formation in patients with a low CHADS2 score receiving warfarin for persistent nonvalvular atrial fibrillation. Cardiovasc Ultrasound 2012;10:50.)

was seen in patients with LV dysfunction even in the absence of AF,[41,42] which suggests that intact LV function may help decrease the risk of thromboembolism.

Local Prothrombotic Agents

Oxidative stress and free radicals
In animal models, induction of AF resulted in a 3-fold increase in the production of superoxide free radicals because of upregulation of xanthine oxidase and nicotinamide adenine dinucleotide phosphate oxidase enzymes.[43] In addition, AF decreases the expression of nitric oxide synthase and thereby decreases nitric oxide production, which is a powerful antithrombotic agent and prevents platelet aggregation.[44] It is therefore possible that decreased nitric oxide in addition to increased free radicals may increase thrombotic milieu. Decreased expression of nitric oxide is associated with increased expression of

prothrombotic plasminogen activator inhibitor type-1 protein in the LA endocardium in AF, but this protein was not found to be increased in LAA.[44]

Adhesion molecules and other procoagulants
Increased expression of adhesion molecules such as intercellular adhesion molecule 1 (ICAM-1) and P-selectin in the LAA were observed in animal models when they were paced to be in AF.[45] Besides, tissue factor expression was also increased in acute AF.[46,47] Anticoagulants such as thrombomodulin and tissue factor pathway inhibitor were downregulated in the atrial endocardium in animal models during AF.[48] Altered procoagulant and anticoagulant factors in AF may therefore tilt the balance toward thrombus formation in the LAA.

von Willebrand factor
It causes platelet adhesion to the endothelial lining. During atrial remodeling in AF, von Willebrand

factor (vWF) is expressed on the endocardial lining.[49,50] Ammash and colleagues[51] validated this finding in patients with nonvalvular AF; vWF antigen and activity levels varied directly with the presence and intensity of SEC and LAA thrombus.

Renin angiotensin system
A few studies have reported an increase in local expression of angiotensin-converting enzyme in atria with AF.[52,53] Angiotensin II induces the Erk class of protein kinases, which in turn activate the fibroblasts and cause interstitial fibrosis resulting in atrial dysfunction.[52] In addition, angiotensin II promotes activation of several other proinflammatory cytokines, such as interleukin-6, tumor necrosis factor alpha, adhesion molecules, thromboxane A2, and metalloproteinases.[22] These proinflammatory cytokines cause endothelial dysfunction and, in association with prothrombotic agents, may result in thrombus formation, especially where the anatomy is suitable, like in the LAA.

Systemic Factors

Platelets
A few studies have reported evidence of increased markers of platelet activation such as β-thromboglobulin, soluble P-selectin, and platelet microparticles in AF.[54,55] In other studies, there was no difference in markers of platelet activation in those with and without AF.[56] Therefore, the role of platelets in LAA thrombus is unclear and needs further investigation.

Procoagulants, growth factors, and cytokines
Plasma fibrinogen levels are increased in acute AF.[46,47] Increased lipoprotein (a) levels have also been associated with thrombus formation in non-valvular chronic AF.[57,58] Lipoprotein (a) contains apolipoprotein, which has a structural homology to plasminogen and therefore this can promote thrombus formation.[57,58] Fibrin D-dimer levels are significantly higher in patients with permanent AF compared with those with paroxysmal AF and normal controls.[46,56] Negative predictive value of D-dimer was 97% for a cutoff level of 1.15 μg/mL.[59] Vascular endothelial growth factor, tissue factor, transforming growth factor beta-1 levels, and angiopoietin 2 levels are all increased in AF.[60,61] It is thought that some of these factors are released in response to mechanical stretch from the atrial tachyarrhythmias.[61]

Others
A lower mean corpuscular volume was associated with higher red cell distribution width and this combination of patients had a higher prevalence of SEC and LAA thrombus; the exact mechanism by which thrombus formation occurs in this case is unclear.[62] Acute onset of AF increases the hematocrit because of the release of atrial natriuretic peptide from LAA and therefore promotes stasis in LAA.[46] A BNP level greater than or equal to 500 pg/mL was associated with thrombus formation in the LAA.[63]

SUMMARY

Thrombus formation in the LAA is caused by the complex interplay of anatomic and histologic changes in the LAA combined with the altered procoagulant state during AF. Therefore assessment of LAA anatomy and function may be considered in addition to $CHADS_2$ and CHA_2DS_2-Vasc to estimate the risk of thromboembolism and the need for anticoagulation in AF. Knowledge about LAA anatomy is also important when patients are being considered for LAA ligation and closure devices.

REFERENCES

1. Di Biase L, Burkhardt JD, Mohanty P, et al. Left atrial appendage: an underrecognized trigger site of atrial fibrillation. Circulation 2010;122(2):109–18.
2. Blackshear JL, Odell JA. Appendage obliteration to reduce stroke in cardiac surgical patients with atrial fibrillation. Ann Thorac Surg 1996;61(2):755–9.
3. Martinsen B, Lohr J. Cardiac development. In: Iaizzo P, editor. Handbook of cardiac anatomy, physiology, and devices. New York: Humana Press; 2005. p. 15–23.
4. Abdulla R, Blew GA, Holterman MJ. Cardiovascular embryology. Pediatr Cardiol 2004;25(3):191–200.
5. Sadler TW. Cardiovascular System. In: Sadler TW, editor. Langman's medical embryology. 11th edition. Philadelphia: Lippincott Williams & Wilkins; 2009.
6. Al-Saady NM, Obel OA, Camm AJ. Left atrial appendage: structure, function, and role in thromboembolism. Heart 1999;82(5):547–54.
7. Ho SY, Anderson RH, Sanchez-Quintana D. Atrial structure and fibres: morphologic bases of atrial conduction. Cardiovasc Res 2002;54(2):325–36.
8. Wang Y, Di Biase L, Horton RP, et al. Left atrial appendage studied by computed tomography to help planning for appendage closure device placement. J Cardiovasc Electrophysiol 2010;21(9):973–82.
9. Ho SY, Cabrera JA, Sanchez-Quintana D. Left atrial anatomy revisited. Circ Arrhythm Electrophysiol 2012;5(1):220–8.
10. Veinot JP, Harrity PJ, Gentile F, et al. Anatomy of the normal left atrial appendage: a quantitative study

of age-related changes in 500 autopsy hearts: implications for echocardiographic examination. Circulation 1997;96(9):3112–5.

11. Di Biase L, Santangeli P, Anselmino M, et al. Does the left atrial appendage morphology correlate with the risk of stroke in patients with atrial fibrillation? Results from a multicenter study. J Am Coll Cardiol 2012;60(6):531–8.

12. Ho SY, McCarthy KP. Anatomy of the left atrium for interventional electrophysiologists. Pacing Clin Electrophysiol 2010;33(5):620–7.

13. Keith A. An account of the structures concerned in the production of the jugular pulse. J Anat Physiol 1907;42(Pt 1):1–25.

14. Miller JP, Albert J, Perrino C, et al. A practical approach to transesophageal echocardiography. 1st edition. Philadelphia: Lippincott Williams & Wilkins; 2003. Common Artifacts and Pitfalls of Clinical Echocardiography.

15. Su P, McCarthy KP, Ho SY. Occluding the left atrial appendage: anatomical considerations. Heart 2008; 94(9):1166–70.

16. Lannigan RA, Zaki SA. Ultrastructure of the myocardium of the atrial appendage. Br Heart J 1966;28(6):796–807.

17. Chapeau C, Gutkowska J, Schiller PW, et al. Localization of immunoreactive synthetic atrial natriuretic factor (ANF) in the heart of various animal species. J Histochem Cytochem 1985;33(6): 541–50.

18. Hara H, Virmani R, Holmes DR, et al. Is the left atrial appendage more than a simple appendage? Catheter Cardiovasc Interv 2009;74(2):234–42.

19. Park HC, Shin J, Ban JE, et al. Left atrial appendage: morphology and function in patients with paroxysmal and persistent atrial fibrillation. Int J Cardiovasc Imaging 2013;29(4):935–44.

20. Frustaci A, Chimenti C, Bellocci F, et al. Histological substrate of atrial biopsies in patients with lone atrial fibrillation. Circulation 1997;96(4):1180–4.

21. Shirani J, Alaeddini J. Structural remodeling of the left atrial appendage in patients with chronic nonvalvular atrial fibrillation: implications for thrombus formation, systemic embolism, and assessment by transesophageal echocardiography. Cardiovasc Pathol 2000;9(2):95–101.

22. Watson T, Shantsila E, Lip GY. Mechanisms of thrombogenesis in atrial fibrillation: Virchow's triad revisited. Lancet 2009;373(9658):155–66.

23. Goldman ME, Pearce LA, Hart RG, et al. Pathophysiologic correlates of thromboembolism in nonvalvular atrial fibrillation: I. Reduced flow velocity in the left atrial appendage (The Stroke Prevention in Atrial Fibrillation [SPAF-III] study). J Am Soc Echocardiogr 1999;12(12):1080–7.

24. Ono K, Iwama M, Kawasaki M, et al. Motion of left atrial appendage as a determinant of thrombus

25. Gage BF, Waterman AD, Shannon W, et al. Validation of clinical classification schemes for predicting stroke: results from the National Registry of Atrial Fibrillation. JAMA 2001;285(22):2864–70.

26. Lip GY, Nieuwlaat R, Pisters R, et al. Refining clinical risk stratification for predicting stroke and thromboembolism in atrial fibrillation using a novel risk factor-based approach: the Euro Heart Survey on Atrial Fibrillation. Chest 2010;137(2):263–72.

27. Beinart R, Heist EK, Newell JB, et al. Left atrial appendage dimensions predict the risk of stroke/TIA in patients with atrial fibrillation. J Cardiovasc Electrophysiol 2011;22(1):10–5.

28. Burrell LD, Horne BD, Anderson JL, et al. Usefulness of left atrial appendage volume as a predictor of embolic stroke in patients with atrial fibrillation. Am J Cardiol 2013;112(8):1148–52.

29. Whisenant BK, Burrell LD, Horne B, et al. Left atrial appendage volume as a predictor of embolic stroke in atrial fibrillation. J Am Coll Cardiol 2013; 61(Suppl 10):E279.

30. Khurram I, Dewire J, Mager M, et al. Role of computed tomography based characteristics of left atrial appendage in predicting risk of stroke in patients with atrial fibrillation. Heart Rhythm 2013; 10(5):S464.

31. Gardner G, Kump J, Chang D, et al. Evaluation of left atrial appendage shape variations in atrial fibrillation patients with stroke. Heart Rhythm 2013;10(5):S464.

32. Agmon Y, Khandheria BK, Gentile F, et al. Echocardiographic assessment of the left atrial appendage. J Am Coll Cardiol 1999;34(7):1867–77.

33. Akoum N, Fernandez G, Wilson B, et al. Association of atrial fibrosis quantified using LGE-MRI with atrial appendage thrombus and spontaneous contrast on transesophageal echocardiography in patients with atrial fibrillation. J Cardiovasc Electrophysiol 2013;24(10):1104–9.

34. Tamura H, Watanabe T, Nishiyama S, et al. Abstract 12932: left atrial strain evaluated by two-dimensional speckle tracking predicts left atrial appendage dysfunction in patients with acute ischemic stroke. Circulation 2012;126(Suppl 21): A12932.

35. Makino N, Nishino M, Ishiyama A, et al. Left atrial appendage morphologic pattern determined by computed tomography is a novel predictor of high risk patient for embolism with atrial fibrillation. J Am Coll Cardiol 2013;61(Suppl 10):E272.

36. Sato C, Tamura H, Watanabe T, et al. Abstract 12993: left atrial dysfunction score evaluated by multiple echocardiographic parameters predicts left atrial appendage thrombus formation in

patients with acute ischemic stroke. Circulation 2012;126(Suppl 21):A12993.

37. Machino-Ohtsuka T, Seo Y, Ishizu T, et al. Significant improvement of left atrial and left atrial appendage function after catheter ablation for persistent atrial fibrillation. Circ J 2013;77(7):1695–704.

38. Yoshida N, Okamoto M, Hirao H, et al. Efficacy of pulmonary vein isolation on left atrial function in paroxysmal and persistent atrial fibrillation and the dependency on its baseline function. Echocardiography 2013;30(7):744–50.

39. Handke M, Harloff A, Hetzel A, et al. Left atrial appendage flow velocity as a quantitative surrogate parameter for thromboembolic risk: determinants and relationship to spontaneous echocontrast and thrombus formation–a transesophageal echocardiographic study in 500 patients with cerebral ischemia. J Am Soc Echocardiogr 2005;18(12):1366–72.

40. Bakalli A, Kamberi L, Pllana E, et al. The influence of left ventricular diameter on left atrial appendage size and thrombus formation in patients with dilated cardiomyopathy. Turk Kardiyol Dern Ars 2010;38(2):90–4.

41. Mahilmaran A, Nayar PG, Sudarsana G, et al. Relationship of left atrial appendage function to left ventricular function. Indian Heart J 2004;56(4):293–8.

42. Agmon Y, Khandheria BK, Gentile F, et al. Clinical and echocardiographic characteristics of patients with left atrial thrombus and sinus rhythm: experience in 20 643 consecutive transesophageal echocardiographic examinations. Circulation 2002;105(1):27–31.

43. Dudley SC Jr, Hoch NE, McCann LA, et al. Atrial fibrillation increases production of superoxide by the left atrium and left atrial appendage: role of the NADPH and xanthine oxidases. Circulation 2005;112(9):1266–73.

44. Cai H, Li Z, Goette A, et al. Downregulation of endocardial nitric oxide synthase expression and nitric oxide production in atrial fibrillation: potential mechanisms for atrial thrombosis and stroke. Circulation 2002;106(22):2854–8.

45. Kamiyama N. Expression of cell adhesion molecules and the appearance of adherent leukocytes on the left atrial endothelium with atrial fibrillation: rabbit experimental model. Jpn Circ J 1998;62(11):837–43.

46. Kamath S, Blann AD, Chin BS, et al. Platelet activation, haemorheology and thrombogenesis in acute atrial fibrillation: a comparison with permanent atrial fibrillation. Heart 2003;89(9):1093–5.

47. Nakamura Y, Nakamura K, Fukushima-Kusano K, et al. Tissue factor expression in atrial endothelia associated with nonvalvular atrial fibrillation: possible involvement in intracardiac thrombogenesis. Thromb Res 2003;111(3):137–42.

48. Yamashita T, Sekiguchi A, Iwasaki YK, et al. Thrombomodulin and tissue factor pathway inhibitor in endocardium of rapidly paced rat atria. Circulation 2003;108(20):2450–2.

49. Fukuchi M, Watanabe J, Kumagai K, et al. Increased von Willebrand factor in the endocardium as a local predisposing factor for thrombogenesis in overloaded human atrial appendage. J Am Coll Cardiol 2001;37(5):1436–42.

50. Kumagai K, Fukuchi M, Ohta J, et al. Expression of the von Willebrand factor in atrial endocardium is increased in atrial fibrillation depending on the extent of structural remodeling. Circ J 2004;68(4):321–7.

51. Ammash N, Konik EA, McBane RD, et al. Left atrial blood stasis and von Willebrand factor-ADAMTS13 homeostasis in atrial fibrillation. Arterioscler Thromb Vasc Biol 2011;31(11):2760–6.

52. Goette A, Staack T, Rocken C, et al. Increased expression of extracellular signal-regulated kinase and angiotensin-converting enzyme in human atria during atrial fibrillation. J Am Coll Cardiol 2000;35(6):1669–77.

53. Dai Y, Wang X, Cao L, et al. Expression of extracellular signal-regulated kinase and angiotensin-converting enzyme in human atria during atrial fibrillation. J Huazhong Univ Sci Technolog Med Sci 2004;24(1):32–6.

54. Choudhury A, Chung I, Blann AD, et al. Elevated platelet microparticle levels in nonvalvular atrial fibrillation: relationship to p-selectin and antithrombotic therapy. Chest 2007;131(3):809–15.

55. Shinohara H, Fukuda N, Soeki T, et al. Relationship between flow dynamics in the left atrium and hemostatic abnormalities in patients with nonvalvular atrial fibrillation. Jpn Heart J 1998;39(6):721–30.

56. Kamath S, Chin BS, Blann AD, et al. A study of platelet activation in paroxysmal, persistent and permanent atrial fibrillation. Blood Coagul Fibrinolysis 2002;13(7):627–36.

57. Igarashi Y, Kasai H, Yamashita F, et al. Lipoprotein(a), left atrial appendage function and thromboembolic risk in patients with chronic nonvalvular atrial fibrillation. Jpn Circ J 2000;64(2):93–8.

58. Igarashi Y, Yamaura M, Ito M, et al. Elevated serum lipoprotein(a) is a risk factor for left atrial thrombus in patients with chronic atrial fibrillation: a transesophageal echocardiographic study. Am Heart J 1998;136(6):965–71.

59. Habara S, Dote K, Kato M, et al. Prediction of left atrial appendage thrombi in non-valvular atrial fibrillation. Eur Heart J 2007;28(18):2217–22.

60. Chung NA, Belgore F, Li-Saw-Hee FL, et al. Is the hypercoagulable state in atrial fibrillation mediated by vascular endothelial growth factor? Stroke 2002;33(9):2187–91.

61. Seko Y, Nishimura H, Takahashi N, et al. Serum levels of vascular endothelial growth factor and transforming growth factor-beta1 in patients with atrial fibrillation undergoing defibrillation therapy. Jpn Heart J 2000;41(1):27–32.

62. Providencia R, Ferreira MJ, Goncalves L, et al. Mean corpuscular volume and red cell distribution width as predictors of left atrial stasis in patients with non-valvular atrial fibrillation. Am J Cardiovasc Dis 2013;3(2):91–102.

63. Doukky R, Gage H, Nagarajan V, et al. B-type natriuretic peptide predicts left atrial appendage thrombus in patients with nonvalvular atrial fibrillation. Echocardiography 2013;30(8):889–95.

Rationale for Left Atrial Appendage Exclusion

Ted Feldman, MD, FESC, FACC, FSCAI

KEYWORDS

- Left atrial appendage • Oral anticoagulant therapy • Warfarin • Atrial fibrillation

KEY POINTS

- The left atrial appendage (LAA) is the source of most systemic emboli in patients with atrial fibrillation (AF), with a cumulative stroke risk greater than 30% over a decade.
- Oral anticoagulant therapy reduces stroke risk by two-thirds.
- Oral anticoagulants are complicated by a relentless major bleeding rate of about 3%/y and intolerance in a significant number of patients.
- New oral agents have advantages over warfarin but are still associated with bleeding and drug intolerance.
- Device therapy for atrial appendage ligation or occlusion is an alternative to drug therapy, without the cumulative incidence of bleeding or the need for anticoagulation.

INTRODUCTION

It has been recognized for decades that the LAA is the source of systemic emboli in patients with AF. The earliest observations were in patients with rheumatic valve disease. In one of the earliest, if not the first, report of resection of the LAA, the investigators note that after an embolus occurs, recurrences are frequent and often fatal. They state, "Since a thrombus is the precursor of every arterial embolus, the ideal prophylaxis for recurrent arterial emboli should be the removal of the thrombus together with its site of origin." The researchers go on to report 2 cases, one of whom survived the operation.[1] A subsequent report described the *notable absence* of recurrent emboli after removal of the auricular appendage.[2]

In the more than half century since these early reports of surgical LAA excision, the authors have added considerable detail to our understanding of the rationale for LAA exclusion. These details constitute the subject of this article.

STROKE AND AF

Cerebrovascular disease is the most common cause of stroke, accounting for 50% to 60% of total stroke.[3] At least 15% of strokes are caused by overt AF, accounting for 75,000 to 1,000,000 embolic strokes each year in the United States.[4–6] Additional patients with subclinical AF may constitute another group with significantly increased stroke risk.[7] The prevalence of stroke increases from 0.1% among adults younger than 55 years to 9.0% in persons 80 years or older. The burden of stroke from AF is large because of the frequency of AF in the US population. At present, there are more than 2 million adults in the United States with AF.[8] The incidence and prevalence of AF is escalating, with the number of AF cases doubling in the next several decades. The lifetime risk for development of AF is approximately 25% among men and women 40 years or older, and this incidence increases with age. At age less than 65 years, the annual stroke rate is about 5%, and this increases to over 8% per year beyond age 75 years.[9] While it is common to characterize stroke risk among patients with AF as a function of percent risk per year, it is sobering to consider aggregate stroke risk. Although the annual rate may be in the range of 3% to 5% per year, about one-third of the patients with AF will have a stroke within 10 years if left untreated.

Disclosure: Dr T. Feldman is a consultant for and receives research grant support from Boston Scientific.
Cardiology Division, Evanston Hospital, NorthShore University HealthSystem, Walgreen Building 3rd Floor, 2650 Ridge Avenue, Evanston, IL 60201, USA
E-mail address: tfeldman@tfeldman.org

Intervent Cardiol Clin 3 (2014) 203–208
http://dx.doi.org/10.1016/j.iccl.2013.11.003

interventional.theclinics.com

AF and LAA Thrombus

It is clear that AF is an important risk factor for stroke. It has been known for many years that the substrate for this risk is LAA thrombus. About 90% of the thrombi responsible for embolic stroke in patients with AF arises from the LAA.[10] This finding comes form a review of reports of over 4700 patients with AF in whom thrombus was detected with transesophageal echo (TEE), at surgery, or at autopsy. Thrombi were present in the LAA and extended into the left atrium (LA) cavity in 57% of patients with rheumatic AF. In contrast, 91% of nonrheumatic-AF-related LA thrombi were isolated to the LAA. There is an enormous surface area for clot to form within the pectinate muscles of the LAA. TEE shows microthrombi in the left atrium of 10% of patients with nonvalvular AF. As many as 20% to 40% of patients with recent thromboemboli have LA clots. Clinically significant thrombi may be 2 to 3 mm in diameter or even smaller.[11]

Assessing Stroke Risk

The use of the CHADS2 stroke risk score, and more recently the CHADS2-VASc score, allows stroke risk stratification for patients with AF (**Table 1**). The CHADS2 was originally based on a group of 1733 patients with AF formed by assigning 1 point each for the presence of congestive heart failure, hypertension, age 75 years or more, and diabetes mellitus and by assigning 2 points for history of stroke or transient ischemic attack.[12] One of the major values of the score is to help identify patients with AF who are at low risk for stroke even without warfarin therapy. The CHADS2 score is a simple, rapid method for risk assessment and allows immediate risk stratification. The CHA2DS2-VASc score further refines the CHADS2 approach by adding further emphasis to female gender and coronary and vascular disease. This score is based on a point system in which 2 points are assigned for a history of stroke or transient ischemic attack or age 75 years or more and 1 point each is assigned for age 65 to 74 years; a history of hypertension, diabetes, recent cardiac failure, vascular disease (myocardial infarction, complex aortic plaque, and peripheral arterial disease (PAD), including prior revascularization, amputation due to PAD, or angiographic evidence of PAD, etc.); and female gender, resulting in a maximum score of 9 points (**Table 2**).[13]

Antithrombotic Therapy for Stroke Prevention in Nonvalvular AF

The standard stroke prevention therapy for AF is anticoagulation. Anticoagulation with a vitamin K antagonist is recommended in the American Heart Association-American College of Cardiology guidelines for patients with more than one moderate risk factor, including age 75 years or more, hypertension, heart failure, impaired left ventricular systolic function with ejection fraction 35% or less or fractional shortening less than 25%, and diabetes mellitus.[14] The European Society of Cardiology guidelines recommend long-term oral anticoagulation for patients with a CHADS2 score of 2 or more, unless contraindicated. In patients with a CHADS2 score of 0 to 1, it is recommended to

Table 1 CHADS2 score	
CHADS2 Score	**Adjusted Stroke Risk (95% CI) per 100 Patient-Years (%)**
0	1.9 (1.2–3.0)
1	2.8 (2.0–3.8)
2	4.0 (3.1–5.1)
3	5.9 (4.6–7.3)
4	8.5 (6.3–11.1)
5	12.5 (8.2–17.5)
6	18.2 (10.5–27.4)

Abbreviation: CI, confidence interval.
Data from Gage BF, Waterman AD, Shannon W, et al. Validation of clinical classification schemes for predicting stroke: results from the National Registry of Atrial Fibrillation. JAMA 2001;285(22):2864–70.

Table 2 CHA2DS2-VASc score	
CHA2DS2-VASc Score	**Rate of Hospital Admission and Death due to Thromboembolism per 100 Person-Years (%)**
0	0.8
1	2
2	3.7
3	5.9
4	9.3
5	15.3
6	19.7
7	21.5
8	22.4
9	23.6

Data from Olesen JB, Lip GY, Hansen ML, et al. Validation of risk stratification schemes for predicting stroke and thromboembolism in patients with atrial fibrillation: nationwide cohort study. BMJ 2011;342:d124.

use a more comprehensive risk-factor-based approach, using the CHA2DS2-VASc score.[13] The relative stroke risk reduction from antithrombotic therapy with vitamin K antagonists is about two-thirds, with an absolute risk reduction of more than 2.5%.[15] This level of stroke risk reduction represents the standard of care in AF.

Limitations of Antithrombotic Therapy for Stroke Prevention in AF

There are several important limitations of antithrombotic agents. It is obvious that any effective anticoagulant treatment will be complicated by bleeding. For warfarin, a significant proportion of patients are out of target range international normalized ratio (INR) at any given time. Unfortunately, there are also a significant number of patients who do not take this therapy, even when it has been recommended.

Bleeding

Intracranial hemorrhage is the most serious bleeding complication. Rates of intracerebral hemorrhage are typically between 0.1% and 0.6% in contemporary reports. Intracranial bleeding increases with INR values 3.5 to 4.0, and there is no increment in bleeding risk with INR values between 2.0 and 3.0 compared with lower INR levels.[16] The annual incidence of anticoagulant-associated intracerebral hemorrhage per 100,000 persons was 0.8 in 1988, 1.9 in 1993/1994, and 4.4 in 1999.[17] Among persons 80 years or older, the anticoagulant-associated intracerebral hemorrhage rate increased from 2.5 in 1988 to 45.9 in 1999! Warfarin distribution in the United States quadrupled on a per capita basis in this time period. Thus, the incidence of anticoagulant-associated intracerebral hemorrhage quintupled in our population during the 1990s. Most of this change can be explained by increasing warfarin use.

In the AFFIRM trial, almost 10% of patients had at least one major bleeding episode over 3.5 years of follow-up.[18] Major bleeding (defined as any central nervous system bleeding or bleeding that required transfusion of 2 or more units of blood, hospitalization in an intensive care unit, and/or discontinuation of anticoagulant or antiplatelet therapy) occurred with an annual incidence of approximately 2% per year. Increased age, heart failure, hepatic or renal disease, diabetes, first AF episode, warfarin use, and aspirin use were significantly associated with major bleeding. The median INR at the time of major bleeding was 2.6, indicating that bleeding is an unavoidable occurrence with warfarin therapy. Minor bleeding (hematuria, gastrointestinal [GI] bleeding, epistaxis, and other reported bleedings that did

not meet the major bleeding criteria listed earlier) was common and occurred in almost 14% of patients. Bleeding is a special problem in patients taking oral anticoagulants undergoing percutaneous coronary intervention. Ordinarily, antiplatelet therapy with aspirin and clopidogrel is indicated. When dual antiplatelet therapy is added to treatment with oral anticoagulants, such triple therapy increases the risk of serious bleeding. A recent report investigated the safety and efficacy of clopidogrel alone compared with clopidogrel plus aspirin in patients on oral anticoagulants. Bleeding episodes were seen in 19.4% patients receiving double therapy and in 44.4% receiving triple therapy. Multiple bleeding events were 6 times more frequent in the triple therapy group (12% vs 2.2%).[19] Bleeding is more common with advancing age. In one prior study, the cumulative incidences of major bleeding at 1, 12, and 48 months were 3%, 11%, and 22%, respectively. The monthly risk of major bleeding decreased over time, from 3% during the first month of outpatient therapy to 0.3% per month after the first year of therapy. Five independent risk factors for major bleeding—age 65 years or greater, history of stroke, history of GI bleeding, a serious comorbid condition (recent myocardial infarction, renal insufficiency, or severe anemia), AF—predicted major bleeding. The cumulative incidence of major bleeding at 48 months was 2% in 57 low-risk patients, 17% in 110 middle-risk patients, and 63% in 20 high-risk patients.[20] Not surprisingly, among patients in whom warfarin is discontinued because of GI bleeding, there is a subsequent high incidence of stroke (5.5%) and death (20%) within 90 days.[21] Older patients have greater bleeding risks, with drug-drug interactions, changing diets, as well as intercurrent illnesses, inherent difficulties, and inconvenience associated with warfarin use.[22]

The bottom line is that bleeding occurs at a relentless rate of about 3% per year in oral-anticoagulant-treated patients with AF.[23]

Untreated and out-of-target-range patients

Many patients never receive oral anticoagulant therapy, and many of those who are treated are often out of therapeutic range. As many as 60% of eligible patients may never be treated.[24] One review of 8 randomized trials encompassed over 55,000 patient-years. On average, patients stayed within the INR range of 2.0 to 3.0 for about 60% to 65% of the time in these controlled clinical trials.[25] Real life studies suggest that this may be as low as 50%. Being below the therapeutic range for more than 60% of the time may completely offset the benefit of this therapy.[26] A population study of AF found that 73% of patients with newly detected AF had some kind of antithrombotic use after AF onset. Among the 76% who were at high risk for stroke, 59% used warfarin, 28% were undertreated with aspirin, and 24% had no therapy (**Fig. 1**).[27] Several studies have suggested that warfarin is prescribed to only two-thirds of individuals with AF who are eligible for anticoagulation.[28] Medication adherence may be a greater problem than with other medicines, because of the need for INR testing.[29]

Alternatives to Warfarin

Oral anticoagulation began with the vitamin K antagonist dicoumarol in 1940. Warfarin was created soon thereafter. These agents produce an anticoagulant effect by interfering with the synthesis of the vitamin-K-dependent clotting factors. An oral direct thrombin inhibitor, the prodrug dabigatran etexilate, was approved in 2010 in the United States for stroke prevention in nonvalvular AF. Two additional agents, rivaroxaban and apixaban are now available, and others such as edoxaban are on the horizon. The major advantage of the new agents is the lack of need for frequent monitoring or dose adjustments. The new oral direct thrombin and factor Xa inhibitors have variations in dosing, half-life, elimination, monitoring, and reversal. These newer agents have lower bleeding rates, particularly hemorrhagic stroke rates, than warfarin (**Table 3**).[30–32] However, the clinical impact of these differences may be more numerically and less clinically important. Also, real life bleeding rates may be much higher than those reported in trials, and approached 9% per year in one recent report.[33] They are further limited by

intolerance, lack of reversibility, and expense compared to warfarin.[34] There are no direct comparisons between dabigatran, rivaroxaban, and apixaban, so assessing their relative merits or deficiencies remains problematic.

What is clear is that with any antithrombotic drug, bleeding will always be an important complication. If we consider warfarin to be problematic, the success of the newer agents is to be possibly less problematic.

Rationale for LAA Exclusion

It has been recognized that the LAA is the principal nidus for thromboembolic stroke among patients with AF for over half a century.[1] Oral anticoagulant therapy with warfarin is the standard of care and reduces stroke risk by two-thirds. Unfortunately, oral anticoagulant therapy has several important limitations, most important among them being bleeding. Major bleeding occurs at a relentless rate of about 3% per year among patients taking warfarin, with a cumulative incidence of 10% to 20% in 3 to 4 years of treatment. A device therapy that eliminates the LAA anatomically has the potential to reduce stroke risk without the ongoing bleeding risks associated with oral anticoagulant therapy. Furthermore, permanent elimination of the LAA by occlusion or ligation will also eliminate the oral anticoagulant problems of time in and out of therapeutic range, the need for anticoagulant interruption for surgical procedures, multiple drug interactions, and drug intolerance due to side effects. Despite the efficacy of oral anticoagulant therapy, there remains an important group of patients who cannot tolerate anticoagulation because of bleeding. An LAA ablative therapy is

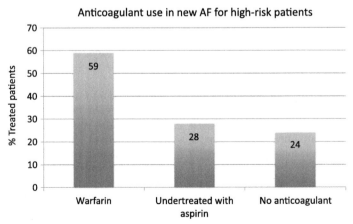

Fig. 1. A population study of AF found that 73% of patients with newly detected AF had some kind of antithrombotic use after AF onset. Among the 76% who were at high risk for stroke, 59% used warfarin, 28% were undertreated with aspirin, and 24% had no therapy. (*Data from* Glazer NL, Dublin S, Smith NL, et al. Newly detected atrial fibrillation and compliance with antithrombotic guidelines. Arch Intern Med 2007;167(3):246–52.)

Table 3
Bleeding rates of newer anticoagulant agents

Study	Treatment	Major Bleeding (%)	Hemorrhagic Stroke (%)
RELY[30]	Dabigatran (110 mg)	2.71	0.12
	Dabigatran (150 mg)	3.11	0.10
	Warfarin	3.36	0.38
ROCKET-AF[31]	Rivaroxaban	3.6	0.5
	Warfarin	3.4	0.7
ARISTOTLE[32]	Apixaban	2.13	0.24
	Warfarin	3.09	0.47

potentially the only alternative for this group. The trade-offs are of course the procedure-related complication rate for a ligation or occlusion therapy and its effectiveness at completely closing the LAA. This balance is easier to achieve in patients with limited or no options for oral anticoagulant therapy. Interestingly, surgical LAA ligation has not clearly been effective enough to sway this balance, because of incomplete LAA exclusion in a significant number of cases.[35] Device therapy offers a clear option for patients who cannot take oral anticoagulants, and as trials are beginning to indicate, an alternative to oral anticoagulants for patients who can take them.[36,37]

REFERENCES

1. Madden JL. Resection of the left auricular appendix. JAMA 1949;140:769–72.
2. Beal JM, Longmire WP, Leake WH. Resection of the auricular appendages. Ann Surg 1950;132:517–30.
3. Wolf PA, Dawber TR, Thomas HE Jr, et al. Epidemiologic assessment of chronic atrial fibrillation and risk of stroke: the Framingham Study. Neurology 1978;28:973–7.
4. Wolf PA, Abbot RD, Kannel WB. Atrial fibrillation: a major contributor to stroke in the elderly. Arch Intern Med 1987;147:1561–4.
5. Wolf PA, Abbot RD, Kannel WB. Atrial fibrillation as an independent risk factor for stroke: the Framingham Study. Stroke 1991;22:983–8.
6. Petersen P, Godtfredson J. Embolic complications in paroxysmal atrial fibrillation. Stroke 1986;17:622–6.
7. Healey JS, Connolly SJ, Gold MR, et al, ASSERT Investigators. Subclinical atrial fibrillation and the risk of stroke. N Engl J Med 2012;366(2):120–9.
8. Go AS, Hylek EM, Phillips KA, et al. Prevalence of diagnosed atrial fibrillation in adults. JAMA 2001; 285:2370–4.
9. Risk factors for stroke and efficacy of antithrombotic therapy in atrial fibrillation. Analysis of pooled data from five randomized controlled trials. Arch Intern Med 1994;154(13):1449–57.
10. Blackshear JL, Odell JA. Appendage obliteration to reduce stroke in cardiac surgical patients with atrial fibrillation [review] [59 refs]. Ann Thorac Surg 1996; 61(2):755–9.
11. Haines DE, Stewart MT, Barka ND, et al. Microembolism and catheter ablation II: effects of cerebral microemboli injection in a canine model. Circ Arrhythm Electrophysiol 2013;6(1):23–30. http://dx.doi.org/10.1161/CIRCEP.112.973461.
12. Gage BF, Waterman AD, Shannon W, et al. Validation of clinical classification schemes for predicting stroke: results from the National Registry of Atrial Fibrillation. JAMA 2001;285(22):2864–70.
13. Camm AJ, Kirchhof P, Lip GY, et al, European Heart Rhythm Association, European Association for Cardio-Thoracic Surgery. Guidelines for the management of atrial fibrillation: the Task Force for the Management of Atrial Fibrillation of the European Society of Cardiology (ESC). Eur Heart J 2010;31(19):2369–429 [Erratum appears in Eur Heart J 2011;32(9):1172].
14. Fuster V, Ryden LE, Cannom DS, et al, American College of Cardiology/American Heart Association Task Force on Practice Guidelines, European Society of Cardiology Committee for Practice Guidelines, European Heart Rhythm Association, Heart Rhythm Society. ACC/AHA/ESC 2006 Guidelines for the Management of Patients with Atrial Fibrillation: a report of the American College of Cardiology/American Heart Association Task Force on Practice Guidelines and the European Society of Cardiology Committee for Practice Guidelines (Writing Committee to Revise the 2001 Guidelines for the Management of Patients With Atrial Fibrillation): developed in collaboration with the European Heart Rhythm Association and the Heart Rhythm Society. Circulation 2006;114(7):e257–354 [Erratum appears in Circulation 2007;116(6):e138].
15. Hart RG, Pearce LA, Aguilar MI. Meta-analysis: antithrombotic therapy to prevent stroke in patients who have nonvalvular atrial fibrillation. Ann Intern Med 2007;146:857–67.
16. Albers GW, Diener HC, Frison L, et al. Ximelagatran vs. warfarin for stroke prevention in patients with

nonvalvular atrial fibrillation: a randomized trial. JAMA 2005;293:690–8.

17. Flaherty ML, Kissela B, Woo D, et al. The increasing incidence of anticoagulant-associated intracerebral hemorrhage. Neurology 2007;68(2):116–21.

18. DiMarco JP, Flaker G, Waldo AL, et al, AFFIRM Investigators. Factors affecting bleeding risk during anticoagulant therapy in patients with atrial fibrillation: observations from the Atrial Fibrillation Follow-up Investigation of Rhythm Management (AFFIRM) study. Am Heart J 2005;149(4):650–6.

19. Dewilde WJ, Oirbans T, Verheugt FW, et al, WOEST Study Investigators. Use of clopidogrel with or without aspirin in patients taking oral anticoagulant therapy and undergoing percutaneous coronary intervention: an open-label, randomised, controlled trial. Lancet 2013;381(9872):1107–15.

20. Landefeld CS, Goldman L. Major bleeding in out-patients treated with warfarin: incidence and prediction by factors known at the start of outpatient therapy. Am J Med 1989;87(2):144–52.

21. Witt DM, Delate T, Garcia DA, et al. Risk of thromboembolism, recurrent hemorrhage, and death after warfarin therapy interruption for gastrointestinal tract bleeding. Arch Intern Med 2012;172(19):1484–91.

22. Zarraga IG, Kron J. Oral anticoagulation in elderly adults with atrial fibrillation: integrating new options with old concepts. J Am Geriatr Soc 2013;61(1):143–50.

23. Dentali F, Douketis JD, Lim W, et al. Combined aspirin-oral anticoagulant therapy compared with oral anticoagulant therapy alone among patients at risk for cardiovascular disease: a meta-analysis of randomized trials. Arch Intern Med 2007;167(2):117–24.

24. Connolly SJ, Eikelboom J, O'Donnell M, et al. Challenges of establishing new antithrombotic therapies in atrial fibrillation. Circulation 2007;116(4):449–55.

25. Agarwal S, Hachamovitch R, Menon V. Current trial-associated outcomes with warfarin in prevention of stroke in patients with nonvalvular atrial fibrillation: a meta-analysis. Arch Intern Med 2012;172(8):623–31.

26. Go AS, Hylek EM, Chang Y, et al. Anticoagulation therapy for stroke prevention in atrial fibrillation: how well do randomized trials translate into clinical practice? JAMA 2003;290:2685–92.

27. Glazer NL, Dublin S, Smith NL, et al. Newly detected atrial fibrillation and compliance with antithrombotic guidelines. Arch Intern Med 2007;167(3):246–52.

28. Nieuwlaat R, Capucci A, Camm AJ, et al. Atrial fibrillation management: a prospective survey in ESC member countries: The Euro Heart Survey on Atrial Fibrillation. Eur Heart J 2005;26:2422–34.

29. Brown MT, Feldman T. Understanding medication adherence: implications for dual antiplatelet therapy. Wayne (PA): Cardiac Interventions Today; 2012. p. 28–32.

30. Connolly SJ, Ezekowitz MD, Yusuf S, et al, RE-LY Steering Committee and Investigators. Dabigatran versus warfarin in patients with atrial fibrillation. N Engl J Med 2009;361(12):1139–51.

31. Patel MR, Mahaffey KW, Garg J, et al, ROCKET AF Investigators. Rivaroxaban versus warfarin in non-valvular atrial fibrillation. N Engl J Med 2011;365(10):883–91.

32. Granger CB, Alexander JH, McMurray JJ, et al, ARISTOTLE Committees and Investigators. Apixaban versus warfarin in patients with atrial fibrillation. N Engl J Med 2011;365(11):981–92.

33. Parikh V, Chainani V, Howard M, et al. Is dabigatran safe in real life? J Am Coll Cardiol 2012;59(13s1):E602.

34. Dittus C, Ansell J. The evolution of oral anticoagulant therapy. Prim Care 2013;40:109–34.

35. Dawsona AG, Asopab S, Dunning J. Should patients undergoing cardiac surgery with atrial fibrillation have left atrial appendage exclusion? Interact Cardiovasc Thorac Surg 2010;10:306–11.

36. Holmes DR, Reddy VY, Turi ZG, et al, PROTECT AF Investigators. Percutaneous closure of the left atrial appendage versus warfarin therapy for prevention of stroke in patients with atrial fibrillation: a randomised non-inferiority trial. Lancet 2009;374(9689):534–42.

37. Gangireddy SR, Halperin JL, Fuster V, et al. Percutaneous left atrial appendage closure for stroke prevention in patients with atrial fibrillation: an assessment of net clinical benefit. Eur Heart J 2012;33(21):2700–8.

Left Atrial Appendage Closure with Transcatheter-Delivered Devices

Brian Whisenant, MD*, Peter Weiss, MD*

KEYWORDS

- Atrial fibrillation • Left atrial appendage • Stroke • Anticoagulation

KEY POINTS

- A large unmet clinical need persists for safe and efficacious stroke prevention in the setting of atrial fibrillation despite the major advances of the novel anticoagulants.
- The PROTECT AF (WATCHMAN Left Atrial Appendage System for Embolic PROTECTion in Patients with Atrial Fibrillation) and CAP (Continued Access to Protect) trials with 3503 patient-years of follow-up in 1122 device-treated patients have demonstrated statistical and clinical stroke and mortality outcomes that compete favorably with those of warfarin. Left atrial appendage (LAA) closure is an alternative to warfarin for patients with a reason to avoid long-term anticoagulation.
- The low event rates noted consistently in the Watchman trials are markedly less than would be anticipated in the absence of anticoagulation. This finding provides a compelling indication for LAA closure among patients who are deemed at high risk or unsuitable for anticoagulation.
- The ultimate potential of LAA closure to prevent strokes and enhance the quality of life relative to oral anticoagulation is promising. Clinical experience, additional clinical investigation, and new LAA technologies may each enhance the already excellent results observed with the Watchman device (Coherex Medical, Salt Lake City, UT).

INTRODUCTION

Left atrial appendage (LAA) closure with transcatheter-delivered devices is an evolving story of compelling randomized data and the potential to dramatically reduce the incidence of stroke and improve the quality of life among patients with atrial fibrillation (AF). Oral anticoagulation is the standard of care for stroke prevention in AF but falls short of providing an adequate solution to this common threat when considered from both efficacy and safety perspectives. Anticoagulation-associated treatment deficits include major and minor bleeding, a large treatment deficit of patients who either cannot or choose to not take oral anticoagulants, and a persistent risk of ischemic stroke and major adverse cardiovascular events among patients taking oral anticoagulants. The robust series of Watchman device (Coherex Medical, Salt Lake City, UT) trials has demonstrated the Watchman device to provide similar stroke prevention efficacy as warfarin and, by extension, provides proof of concept of LAA closure. Realizing the ultimate potential of LAA closure will demand additional research.

THE ORAL ANTICOAGULATION TREATMENT DEFICIT

The tremendous unmet clinical need for safe and efficacious stroke reduction in patients with AF that persists despite the novel anticoagulants establishes the foundation and motivation for LAA occlusion. AF is a chronic condition. The persistent

Dr B. Whisenant acknowledges a financial interest in Coherex Medical.
Division of Cardiology, Intermountain Medical Center, 5121 South Cottonwood Street, Level 6, Salt Lake City, UT 84157, USA
* Corresponding author.
E-mail addresses: brian.whisenant@imail.org; pete.weiss@imail.org

Intervent Cardiol Clin 3 (2014) 209–218
http://dx.doi.org/10.1016/j.iccl.2014.01.002
2211-7458/14/$ – see front matter

risk of anticoagulant-associated hemorrhage renders chronic anticoagulation inherently undesirable. There are unmet clinical needs for additional stroke prevention among those at high risk for AF-mediated stroke despite anticoagulation,[1] for those at low risk in whom the anticoagulation-associated bleeding risk may not be justified, and for those unable or unwilling to take oral anticoagulants. The large randomized trials comparing the novel anticoagulants with warfarin for the prevention of stroke in AF provide abundant data on both the newer drugs as well as warfarin.[2–5] The annualized rate of stroke and systemic embolism exceeded 1.5% with warfarin and 1.1% with the novel anticoagulants in each of these trials. The annualized risk of major bleeding exceeded 3% with warfarin and 2% with the novel agents. Although these annualized numbers may seem acceptably low at first glance, the chronic, lifelong nature of AF results in sobering levels of stroke over longer-term follow-up. For example, among the patients randomized to high-dose edoxaban in the Engage AF Trial, the annualized rate of stroke or systemic embolism was 1.18%. With a median treatment exposure of 907 days, 4.2% of the high-dose edoxaban patients experienced a stroke or systemic embolism, 11.8% experienced a major adverse cardiac event, 6.0% experienced major bleeding, and 26.6% experienced overt bleeding.[5] Patients with AF considered low or moderate risk with a CHADS2 score of 0 or 1 have a still-concerning annualized stroke rate between 1.8% and 4.0%.[6,7] Oral anticoagulant (OAC) therapy is considered optional according to current American College of Cardiology/American Heart Association guidelines for patients with a CHADS2 score of 1 because of the significant risk of OAC-associated bleeding, which mitigates the benefit of stroke reduction.[8] Although the CHA2DS2-VASc[9] score provides additional risk factor–based stratification, stroke prevention among these lower-risk patients represents yet another unmet clinical need. The persistent risk of stroke, bleeding, and major adverse cardiovascular events despite anticoagulation with even the novel anticoagulants emphasizes the unmet need for effective therapy providing long-term stroke prevention and minimized comorbidity.

In addition to the long-term morbidity and mortality associated with oral anticoagulation, physician prescribing practices and patient compliance limit the benefit of oral anticoagulation. Numerous studies have demonstrated that just more than 50% of high-risk patients with AF are prescribed anticoagulants.[10] Two years after initiating anticoagulation in the RE-LY trial, 17% of patients had discontinued warfarin and 21% had discontinued dabigatran.[3] The novel oral anticoagulants (NOACS) have captured the market share from warfarin but have not yet demonstrated an increase in the overall penetration of anticoagulation among patients at high risk for stroke with AF.[11] The AVERROES trial demonstrated a significant reduction in the primary end point of stroke or systemic embolism with apixaban when compared with aspirin among patients deemed unsuitable for vitamin K antagonist therapy. However, the AVERROES trial specifically excluded patients with a high risk of bleeding including those with documented hemorrhagic tendencies.[10] AVERROES captured primarily a warfarin-unwilling population rather than an anticoagulant-contraindicated population. There remains a tremendous unmet clinical need to reduce stroke among patients with AF who are either not prescribed or unwilling to take oral anticoagulants as directed.

EMERGENCE OF LAA CLOSURE
LAA Surgical Occlusion and Excision

Like many transcatheter procedures and devices, the concept of LAA occlusion originated with surgery. The potential of reducing the risk of AF-mediated stroke through LAA exclusion was first explored surgically before the advent of cardiopulmonary bypass[12] and became a common adjunct to surgery by the 1990s, albeit with less-than-complete exclusion in some cases.[13–15] The benefit of LAA surgical excision may receive its most definitive evidence in the 4700-patient Left Atrial Appendage Occlusion Study III trial, which is now randomizing surgical patients to adjunctive LAA excision or no therapy (clinicaltrials.gov NCT01561651).

Appriva: PLAATO Device

The first percutaneous implantable LAA occluder is largely recognized as the PLAATO device, developed by Appriva Medical (Sunnyvale, CA) (**Fig. 1**). Appriva, founded in 1998, coined the PLAATO procedure (percutaneous left atrial appendage transcatheter occlusion) and initially named their device X-Caliber. Over time it became known as the PLAATO system and device. The PLAATO device is a nitinol self-expanding cage, delivered to the LAA via transcatheter techniques. The left atrial–facing surface is covered with occlusive polytetrafluoroethylene (PTFE). Retention anchors engage the LAA wall. The PLAATO device was evaluated in a series of well-conducted prospective registries.[16,17] Early investigators demonstrated that the PLAATO device did not interfere with pulmonary vein flow or mitral valve function,[18] and postmortem analysis of a

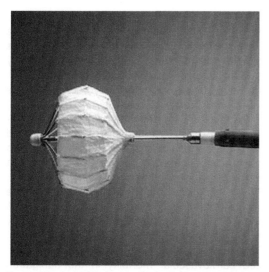

Fig. 1. The PLAATO device. (Copyright © 2014 Boston Scientific Corporation or its affiliates. All rights reserved. Used with permission of the Boston Scientific Corporation.)

patient who died of noncardiac causes 1 year after PLAATO implantation revealed complete device endothelialization without device-associated thrombus.[19] Although the initial PLAATO experience included important complications, including periprocedural death, cardiac tamponade with surgical drainage, and device embolization, most of the procedures were uncomplicated and of relatively short duration. Follow-up transesophageal echocardiography (TEE) interrogation revealed successful closure in most patients, and long-term follow-up of the patients managed with the PLAATO device and aspirin revealed a risk of stroke much less than predicted by the CHADS scoring system with aspirin therapy alone.[17,20] Appriva received CE mark approval in 2002 and was purchased by EV3/Covidien (EV3 Endovascular, Inc, Plymouth, MN) shortly afterward. Appriva and then EV3 explored the possibility of randomizing patients unable to take warfarin between either LAA closure with the PLAATO device or conventional management with aspirin. EV3 found the prospects of this trial to be daunting and, despite a promising initial clinical experience, chose not to initiate a US pivotal trial and did not commercialize the PLAATO device outside of the United States. The Appriva intellectual property was eventually sold to Atritech. The PLAATO experience demonstrated that the LAA could be successfully closed with a transcatheter-delivered implant and provided a foundation for future device development and clinical studies of LAA closure.

DATA-DRIVEN LAA CLOSURE: THE WATCHMAN LAA OCCLUDER

Atritech Medical was founded in 2003 with the Watchman LAA occluder. The Watchman device was initially evaluated in a combined US and European feasibility trial of 75 patients. Despite iterating the Watchman device during this early experience and working through typical first-in-man learning curve issues, 90% of enrolled patients were able to discontinue warfarin; there were no observed strokes during a mean follow-up of 740 days.[21] This initial clinical experience led to the CE mark of the Watchman device in 2005. However, Atritech postponed marketing outside the United States while they focused on completing the US pivotal PROTECT AF trial. Boston Scientific (Natick, MA) purchased Atritech in 2011 and now distributes the Watchman device.

The PROTECT AF trial is the seminal trial proving both the efficacy of the Watchman device as well as the concept of LAA closure. Initiated in 2005, the PROTECT AF trial randomized 707 patients in a 2:1 ratio with 463 randomized to the device and 244 randomized to warfarin therapy with a primary combined end point of all stroke, systemic thromboembolism, and cardiovascular death. The Bayesian statistical plan allowed for sequential evaluation of the patients in increments of 150 patient-years up to 1500 patient-years but then called for ongoing follow-up through 5 years.[22] The trial met its noninferiority primary efficacy end point with an incidence of cardiovascular death, stroke, or systemic embolism of 3.0% with the device and 4.9% with warfarin therapy.[23] The PROTECT AF trial was debated at a Food and Drug Administration (FDA) advisory panel in April 2009. Although the panel voted for approval, the FDA issued a letter of nonapproval in 2010 citing, among other concerns, device- and procedure-associated adverse events, inclusion of moderate-risk $CHADS2 = 1$ patients, and relatively short follow-up.[24] Boston Scientific updated the PROTECT AF data set at the December 2013 FDA panel meeting with 2621 patient-years of follow-up. This most recent analysis revealed a primary efficacy event rate of 2.2 events per 100 patient-years with the device compared with 3.8 events per 100 patient-years with control (posterior probability of superiority = 0.96). The stroke rate among patients randomized to Watchman (1.5 per 100 patient-years) compared favorably with the control (2.2 per 100 patient-years), with a posterior noninferior probability of 0.999.[25]

Atritech enrolled 566 patients with a mean CHADS2 score of 2.5 in the nonrandomized Continued Access to Protect (CAP) registry during the transition from completion of PROTECT AF until they received Food and Drug Administration approval to initiate a the confirmatory Thromboembolic Prevention in Patients with Non-valvular Atrial Fibrillation (PREVAIL) randomized trial. The CAP registry demonstrated improved safety compared with PROTECT AF.[26] The efficacy results were presented at the European Society of Cardiology (ESC) meetings in 2013[27] and reviewed at the December 11, 2013 FDA panel meeting.[25] The CAP primary efficacy end point (stroke, systemic embolism, and cardiovascular death) was observed at a rate of 2.0 events per 100 patient-years (27 events per 1328 patient-years). There were 14 ischemic strokes and 1 hemorrhagic stroke during the 1328 patient-years of follow-up yielding a composite stroke rate of 1.13 strokes per 100 patient-years. When PROTECT AF and CAP were combined to provide 3503 patient-years of follow-up in 1122 device-treated patients, the combined primary end point (stroke, systemic embolism, and cardiovascular death) event rate was 2.14 events per 100 patient-years, and the combined ischemic stroke rate was 1.26 events per 100 patient-years. Although the CAP efficacy data awaits peer-reviewed publication, the absolute event rates compare favorably with the NOAC trials (**Table 1**).

The favorable incidence of cardiovascular mortality in PROTECT AF and CAP when compared with the warfarin and the novel anticoagulants may be considered hypothesis generating and warrants additional investigation (see **Table 1**; **Fig. 2**). Annualized cardiovascular mortality in the device arms of PROTECT AF and CAP was 1.0% and 0.89%, respectively. Cardiovascular mortality in the warfarin arm of PROTECT AF was 2.4%. Despite similar mean CHADS2 scores, the annualized cardiovascular mortality in the dabigatran 150-mg arm of RE-LY was 2.3% and in the apixaban arm of Apixaban arm of Aristotle was 1.8%. The WOEST (What is the Optimal antiplatElet and

Table 1
Stroke, systemic embolism, and cardiovascular mortality for Watchman, novel anticoagulants, and warfarin

	Stroke & Systemic Embolism		Cardiovascular Mortality	
PROTECT AF	Watchman N = 463, CHADS2 = 2.2	Warfarin N = 244, CHADS2 = 2.2	Watchman N = 463, CHADS2 = 2.2	Warfarin N = 244, CHADS2 = 2.2
1065 pt y[23]	2.6	3.2	0.7	2.7
1588 pt y[26]	2.3	2.7	1.0	2.8
2621 pt y[25]	1.7	2.2	1.0	2.4
CAP	Watchman N = 566, CHADS2 = 2.5	—	Watchman N = 566, CHADS2 = 2.5	—
1350 pt y[25]	1.2	—	0.89	—
RE-LY[3]	Dabigatran 150 mg BID N = 6076 CHADS2 = 2.2 1.1	Warfarin N = 6022 CHADS2 = 2.1 1.7	Dabigatran 150 mg BID N = 6076 CHADS2 = 2.2 2.3	Warfarin N = 6022 CHADS2 = 2.1 2.7
ROCKET AF[4]	Rivaroxaban N = 7131 CHADS2 = 3.5 1.7	Warfarin N = 7133 CHADS2 = 3.5 2.2	Rivaroxaban N = 7131 CHADS2 = 3.5 —	Warfarin N = 7133 CHADS2 = 3.5 —
ARISTOTLE[2]	Apixaban N = 9120 CHADS2 = 2.1 1.3	Warfarin N = 9081 CHADS2 = 2.1 1.6	Apixaban N = 9120 CHADS2 = 2.1 1.8	Warfarin N = 9081 CHADS2 = 2.1 2.0
ENGAGE AF[5]	Edoxaban 60 mg N = 7035 CHADS2 = 2.8 1.6	Warfarin N = 7036 CHADS2 = 2.8 1.8	Edoxaban 60 mg N = 7035 CHADS2 = 2.8 2.7	Warfarin N = 7036 CHADS2 = 2.8 3.2

Abbreviations: ARISTOTLE, Apixaban for the Prevention of Stroke in Subjects With Atrial Fibrillation; ENGAGE AF-TIMI 48, The Effective Anticoagulation with Factor Xa Next Generation in Atrial Fibrillation–Thrombolysis in Myocardial Infarction 48; pt, patient; ROCKET AF, The Rivaroxaban Once Daily Oral Direct Factor Xa Inhibition Compared with Vitamin K Antagonism for Prevention of Stroke and Embolism Trial in Atrial Fibrillation.
Data from Refs.[2–5,23,25,26]

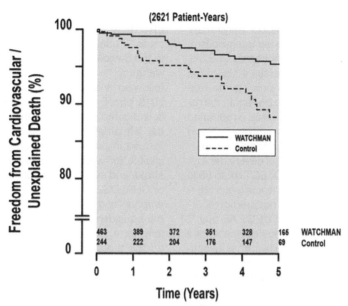

Fig. 2. PROTECT AF: freedom from cardiovascular/unexplained death, Kaplan-Meier curves at 2621 patient-years. (*From* FDA. FDA executive summary: Boston Scientific WATCHMAN Left Atrial Appendage Closure Therapy. Prepared for the December 11, 2013 meeting of the Circulatory System Devices Panel. Available at: http://www.fda.gov/downloads/AdvisoryCommittees/CommitteesMeetingMaterials/MedicalDevices/MedicalDevicesAdvisoryCommittee/CirculatorySystemDevicesPanel/UCM377935.pdf.)

anticoagulant therapy in patients with oral anticoagulation and coronary StenTing) trial randomized coronary stent patients taking anticoagulants to either double therapy with clopidogrel or triple therapy with clopidogrel and aspirin. Although the primary outcome of any bleeding was more common with triple therapy than double therapy (44.4% vs 19.4%, P = .001), the secondary end point of all-cause mortality was also more common with triple therapy (6.3% vs 2.5%, P = .027).[28] Although such comparisons have significant limitations, including the relatively small sample size of the Watchman trials and the potential for adjudication differences, one may hypothesize various mechanisms whereby anticoagulant-associated bleeding may have similarly translated into excess mortality in these various trials.

The PREVAIL trial randomized 407 patients in a 2:1 fashion to the Watchman device (N = 269) and warfarin (N = 138). The PREVAIL Bayesian statistical design incorporated prior patients from PROTECT AF as well as newly randomized patients in PREVAIL while discounting the contribution of the PROTECT AF patients. PREVAIL was designed with 3 coprimary end points. A mechanism of action end point comparing ischemic stroke more than 7 days after Watchman implantation demonstrated noninferiority with warfarin. The safety end point also achieved its performance goal with a low rate of procedural complications. However,

the initial efficacy end point failed to demonstrate statistical noninferiority. The 18-month projected composite rate of stroke, systemic embolism, and cardiovascular death was 0.064 with the device and 0.063 with warfarin. Although this projected event rate was essentially equivalent between Watchman and warfarin, the confidence interval exceeded the prespecified noninferiority margin of 1.75 and, therefore, failed to prove noninferiority.[25] The FDA encouraged its panel members to consider the totality of data when evaluating the Watchman device. The FDA panel voted 13:1 in favor of approval.[29] At the time of this writing, final FDA approval and the associated label remain under FDA consideration.

The Watchman Learning Curve

The PROTECT AF trial was handicapped by the early experience with this technology. Among the 468 patients randomized to LAA closure in the PROTECT AF trial, 408 received devices; warfarin was discontinued in 348 patients at 45 days. The most common reason patients did not receive a device was a failed attempt (N = 41), and the most common reason for continuing warfarin at 45 days was residual flow around the device (N = 30). In a per protocol analysis comparing PROTECT AF patients who were randomized to device, received a device and stopped warfarin per protocol with those who were randomized to warfarin and took warfarin per protocol, the primary composite end point (stroke, systemic embolism, and cardiovascular death) was observed in 2.3% of the device patients per year versus 4.1% of the warfarin patients per year, thus proving the true potential of LAA closure.[30] With experience, the results in the CAP registry demonstrated a reduction in acute procedural complications from 7.7% in PROTECT AF to 3.7% in CAP, whereas the percentage of patients with successful device deployment increased from 87% in PROTECT AF to 95% in CAP.[26] Although residual peri-device leaks adjacent to the Watchman device did not predict recurrent neurologic events in the PROTECT AF trial,[31] the potential to further reduce postdevice stroke through enhanced closure warrants further investigation. Promising results from the next-generation Watchman device Evolve registry were presented in August 2011 at the ESC meetings. However, Boston Scientific continues to iterate this device, and it is not yet commercially available.

Current Indications for LAA Closure

There is some debate regarding the population of patients most appropriately considered for LAA occlusion at this time. The greatest unmet clinical need is arguably among patients who cannot or choose to not take oral anticoagulants. A successful randomized trial comparing LAA closure with antiplatelet therapy or no therapy in patients contraindicated to oral anticoagulants would provide a mandate to treat such patients and definitively demonstrate the efficacy of LAA closure. However, many perceive such a trial to be unethical in light of the overwhelming efficacy of the available Watchman trials. The yearly incidence of AF-mediated stroke without oral anticoagulation is well documented in excess of 5% in both the numerous trials comparing warfarin with aspirin or no therapy[32] as well as the large-scale stroke trials.[6,7] The long-term yearly stroke rate of 1.26% in PROTECT AF and CAP, with 1122 Watchman-allocated patients and 3503 patient-years of follow-up, has demonstrated that the Watchman device not only competes favorably with warfarin but is dramatically less than predicted without oral anticoagulation. The ESC, therefore, seems justified in suggesting that LAA closure be considered for patients with a high stroke risk and contraindications for long-term oral anticoagulation.[33]

The FDA panel seemed to largely support the ESC's guidelines endorsing LAA closure for contraindicated patients while further extending support to those who would prefer to avoid long-term anticoagulation. A quality-of-life substudy of PROTECT AF demonstrated a significantly increased quality of life among patients randomized to the device compared with those randomized to warfarin.[34] Boston Scientific proposed the following indication for use at the December 2013 panel meeting: "Watchman LAAC Therapy is indicated to prevent thromboembolism from the left atrial appendage. It may be considered for use in patients with non-valvular AF who are eligible for warfarin therapy to reduce the risk of stroke and systemic embolism based on CHADS2 or CHA2DS2-VASc scores." The panel suggested emphasizing a personalized approach including the consideration of patient preference regarding long-term anticoagulation therapy and suggested adding the statement "and who have reason not to remain on chronic warfarin therapy"[29] to the end of the current indications for use.

EMERGING LAA INVESTIGATION AND TECHNOLOGIES
Adjunctive Pharmacology

The optimal adjunctive pharmacology both early and late following LAA device closure has varied in clinical trials and warrants additional investigation. Surveillance TEEs in the Watchman trials demonstrated rare device-associated thrombus. Most of these patients did not experience thromboembolic events, and many of these thrombi occurred during interruption of protocol-prescribed medications. The PROTECT AF and PREVAIL trials required 6 weeks of warfarin anticoagulation along with 81 mg of aspirin following device deployment; this was followed by dual antiplatelet therapy with aspirin and clopidogrel until 6 months after device deployment and then indefinite aspirin therapy. The Aspirin Plavix Feasibility Study with Watchman Left Atrial Appendage Closure Technology (ASAP) registry demonstrated that the Watchman device may be safely implanted without a warfarin transition resulting in an ischemic stroke rate less than that expected based on the CHADS2 scores of the patient cohort.[35] The WaveCrest I protocol suggested dual antiplatelet therapy after Coherex WaveCrest (Coherex Medical, Salt Lake City, UT) deployment for 90 days and then aspirin alone. The exception to this guideline was for patients with a history of stroke who were taking oral anticoagulants before WaveCrest implantation who continued anticoagulation until LAA closure was demonstrated at follow-up TEE.

The rate of device endothelialization varies between patients and may vary between devices.[36] Patient phenotype, clinical history, and stroke risk may also influence optimal adjunctive pharmacology. Among the 133 patients with a history of prior stroke randomized in the PROTECT AF trial, the primary efficacy end point favored the Watchman device over warfarin, albeit with wide confidence intervals.[30] Observations of device-associated thrombus have led to suggestions that patients with low ejection fractions or higher CHADS2 scores may be better served with a warfarin transition than dual antiplatelet therapy.[37] Lower-dose anticoagulation with either warfarin or a novel agent in addition to LAA closure may be an effective, albeit expensive, approach to stroke mitigation for patients at the highest risk of recurrent AF-mediated stroke. However, excess thromboembolic events among mechanical heart valve patients randomized to dabigatran when compared with those randomized to warfarin has raised concerns that the novel anticoagulants may not be an appropriate adjunctive option following LAA device closure.[38] It is hoped that the anticipated Watchman device approval will serve as a foundation for additional investigation that will tailor adjunctive pharmacology strategies to individual patients.

AGA Medical/St. Jude Medical: Amplatzer Cardiac Plug

As reports of LAA closure initially surfaced, the Amplatzer Septal Occluder (Amplatzer SO, St. Jude Medical, St Paul, MN), designed for closure of atrial septal defects, was on occasion used in an off-label fashion to close the LAA. This use was generally justified only in patients deemed to be contraindicated to warfarin with a high risk of stroke. Because the SO device relied on radial expansion force without active fixation for anchoring, device embolization was a relatively common complication. AGA adapted their well-established nitinol weave devices with the target of LAA occlusion as the Amplatzer Cardiac Plug (ACP) and obtained CE mark approval with an indication for the closure of cardiac structures in 2008. The published data on the ACP device are limited by retrospective single-center and nonrandomized methodology.[37,39] Although the ACP has extensive commercial use outside the United States, the relative merits of the ACP device compared with the Watchman device remain speculative and anecdotal. The US pivotal AMPLATZER Cardiac Plug Clinical Trial is currently randomizing patients between the ACP device and optimal medical therapy with either warfarin or dabigatran. However, the FDA demanded exclusions, including a history of prior AF ablation; poorly regulated International Normalized Ratio (INR)

have limited enrollment. The next-generation Amulet device was voluntarily withdrawn by St. Jude and is not available commercially at this time.

Emerging Technologies

Numerous next-generation LAA closure technologies are in various stages of development and clinical testing. Both the Watchman and the ACP are associated with limitations that may or may not be improved on with next-generation devices. Opportunities for technology-driven enhanced outcomes include (1) suitability for more anatomies and enhanced closure of the entire LAA; (2) diminished procedural complications, including stroke, tamponade, and device embolization; and (3) improved long-term stroke reduction, which may be a function of completeness of LAA closure and device materials.

The Coherex WaveCrest LAA Occluder

The Coherex WaveCrest LAA occluder separates occlusion and anchoring, is designed to be positioned in the ostium of the LAA, and is constructed with expanded polytetrafluoroethylene (ePTFE) facing the left atrium to minimize thrombus formation (**Fig. 3**). The device is anchored with 20 microtines distributed circumferentially at the distal device margin. Distal anchoring allows the device to be deployed in shallow appendages and proximal to any bifurcation of lobes. Contrast may be injected through the delivery system, beyond the occluder, which assists in the assessment of stability and seal. The WaveCrest I trial conducted in Europe, Australia, and New Zealand enrolled 73 patients with the current-generation device. Acute results presented by Dr Vivek Reddy in the October 2013 Congenital & Structural Interventions (CSI) meeting demonstrated successful deployment in 70 of 73 patients, with core laboratory adjudicated closure in 67 of 69 patients with available TEEs for a 45-day review. The Coherex WaveCrest occlusion system received CE mark approval in August 2013 and is available in select countries through a distribution agreement with Johnson & Johnson. The US pivotal WaveCrest II trial is anticipated in 2014.

Occlutech LAA Occluder

The Occlutech LAA Occluder (Occlutech International AB, Helsingborg, Sweden) is a self-expanding Nitinol wire mesh with "shape-memory" properties that is anchored with closed loops at the distal device margin (**Fig. 4**). The closed loops are designed to engage the trabeculated LAA while avoiding LAA perforation and tamponade. The conical shape of the occluder tapers distally

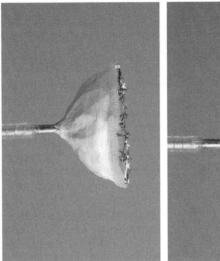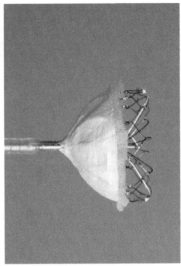

Fig. 3. The Coherex WaveCrest LAA occluder. (*Courtesy of* Coherex Medical, Salt Lake City, UT; with permission.)

from the LAA ostium, thereby providing adaptable radial expansion force. The polymer covering seals the LAA with deployment and serves as a scaffold for endothelialization. A ball-shaped connection hub allows the occluder to pivot relative to the delivery system.

LifeTech LAA Occluder: LAmbre

The LifeTech LAmbre LAA occluder (Lifetech Scientific, Shenzhen, China) consists of an LA cover

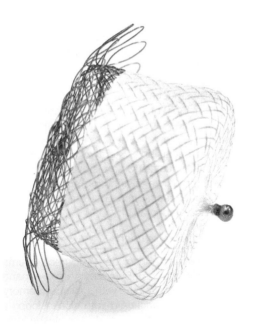

Fig. 4. The Occlutech LAA occluder. (*Courtesy of* Occlutech International AB, Helsingborg, Sweden; with permission.)

and a distal umbrella anchor joined by a short central waist. The umbrella anchor has a combination of distal ball-tipped frames with sidewall hooks. A successful 19-patient Asian registry was completed in 2013 while a CE mark study was initiated with early promising results.[40]

Cardia Ultrasept LAA Occluder

The Cardia Ultrasept LAA Occluder (Cardia Inc, Eagan, MN) consists of a soft left atrium–facing sail manufactured from polyvinyl alcohol and a distal bulb for anchoring the device. An articulating technology between the anchor bulb and the proximal sail allows the occluder to conform to tortuous anatomies. The distal anchor includes lateral wall hooks. The Ultrasept LAA device is fully retrievable. The initial human experience in Brazil was reported as promising.

SUMMARY

The persistent incidence of AF-related stroke and anticoagulation-associated bleeding despite recent advances in anticoagulation pharmacology leaves a tremendous unmet need for enhanced and safer stroke prevention among patients with AF. The remarkably successful Watchman trials have demonstrated that the Watchman device competes favorably with warfarin in terms of stroke and cardiovascular mortality. The low stroke rate of patients receiving the Watchman device compared with historical rates of stroke among patients treated with aspirin or no therapy creates a compelling option for patients unable or unwilling to take oral anticoagulants. LAA closure is now an option for patients with a reason not to take anticoagulants. Procedural experience, iterative technologies, and expanding understanding of adjunctive pharmacology may enhance the outcomes of LAA closure. The current Watchman trials and anticipated FDA approval will launch additional investigation that will help define the ultimate potential of LAA closure to prevent strokes and enhance the quality of life relative to oral anticoagulation.

REFERENCES

1. Lip GY, Frison L, Halperin JL, et al. Identifying patients at high risk for stroke despite anticoagulation: a comparison of contemporary stroke risk stratification schemes in an anticoagulated atrial fibrillation cohort. Stroke 2010;41(12):2731–8.
2. Granger CB, Alexander JH, McMurray JJ, et al. Apixaban versus warfarin in patients with atrial fibrillation. N Engl J Med 2011;365(11):981–92.
3. Connolly SJ, Ezekowitz MD, Yusuf S, et al. Dabigatran versus warfarin in patients with atrial fibrillation. N Engl J Med 2009;361(12):1139–51.
4. Patel MR, Mahaffey KW, Garg J, et al. Rivaroxaban versus warfarin in nonvalvular atrial fibrillation. N Engl J Med 2011;365(10):883–91.
5. Giugliano RP, Ruff CT, Braunwald E, et al. Edoxaban versus warfarin in patients with atrial fibrillation. N Engl J Med 2013;369(22):2093–104.
6. Gage BF, Waterman AD, Shannon W, et al. Validation of clinical classification schemes for predicting stroke: results from the National Registry of Atrial Fibrillation. JAMA 2001;285(22):2864–70.
7. Gage BF, van Walraven C, Pearce L, et al. Selecting patients with atrial fibrillation for anticoagulation: stroke risk stratification in patients taking aspirin. Circulation 2004;110(16):2287–92.
8. Anderson JL, Halperin JL, Albert NM, et al. Management of patients with atrial fibrillation (compilation of 2006 ACCF/AHA/ESC and 2011 ACCF/AHA/HRS recommendations): a report of the American College of Cardiology/American Heart Association Task Force on Practice Guidelines. J Am Coll Cardiol 2013;61(18):1935–44.
9. Lip GY, Nieuwlaat R, Pisters R, et al. Refining clinical risk stratification for predicting stroke and thromboembolism in atrial fibrillation using a novel risk factor-based approach: the euro heart survey on atrial fibrillation. Chest 2010;137(2):263–72.
10. Connolly SJ, Eikelboom J, Joyner C, et al. Apixaban in patients with atrial fibrillation. N Engl J Med 2011; 364(9):806–17.
11. Kirley K, Qato DM, Kornfield R, et al. National trends in oral anticoagulant use in the United States, 2007 to 2011. Circ Cardiovasc Qual Outcomes 2012; 5(5):615–21.
12. Madden JL. Resection of the left auricular appendix; a prophylaxis for recurrent arterial emboli. J Am Med Assoc 1949;140(9):769–72.
13. Blackshear JL, Odell JA. Appendage obliteration to reduce stroke in cardiac surgical patients with atrial fibrillation. Ann Thorac Surg 1996;61(2):755–9.
14. Lynch M, Shanewise JS, Chang GL, et al. Recanalization of the left atrial appendage demonstrated by transesophageal echocardiography. Ann Thorac Surg 1997;63(6):1774–5.
15. Kanderian AS, Gillinov AM, Pettersson GB, et al. Success of surgical left atrial appendage closure: assessment by transesophageal echocardiography. J Am Coll Cardiol 2008;52(11):924–9.
16. Sievert H, Lesh MD, Trepels T, et al. Percutaneous left atrial appendage transcatheter occlusion to prevent stroke in high-risk patients with atrial fibrillation: early clinical experience. Circulation 2002;105(16):1887–9.
17. Ostermayer SH, Reisman M, Kramer PH, et al. Percutaneous left atrial appendage transcatheter occlusion (PLAATO system) to prevent stroke in high-risk patients with non-rheumatic atrial fibrillation: results from the international multi-center feasibility trials. J Am Coll Cardiol 2005;46(1):9–14.
18. Hanna IR, Kolm P, Martin R, et al. Left atrial structure and function after percutaneous left atrial appendage transcatheter occlusion (PLAATO): six-month echocardiographic follow-up. J Am Coll Cardiol 2004;43(10):1868–72.
19. Omran H, Schmidt H, Hardung D, et al. Post mortem analysis of a left atrial appendage occlusion device (PLAATO) in a patient with permanent atrial fibrillation. J Interv Card Electrophysiol 2005;14(1):17–20.
20. Block PC, Burstein S, Casale PN, et al. Percutaneous left atrial appendage occlusion for patients in atrial fibrillation suboptimal for warfarin therapy: 5-year results of the PLAATO (Percutaneous Left Atrial Appendage Transcatheter Occlusion) study. JACC Cardiovasc Interv 2009;2(7):594–600.
21. Sick PB, Schuler G, Hauptmann KE, et al. Initial worldwide experience with the WATCHMAN left atrial appendage system for stroke prevention in atrial fibrillation. J Am Coll Cardiol 2007;49(13):1490–5.
22. Fountain RB, Holmes DR, Chandrasekaran K, et al. The PROTECT AF (WATCHMAN Left Atrial Appendage System for Embolic PROTECTion in Patients with Atrial Fibrillation) trial. Am Heart J 2006; 151(5):956–61.
23. Holmes DR, Reddy VY, Turi ZG, et al. Percutaneous closure of the left atrial appendage versus warfarin therapy for prevention of stroke in patients with atrial fibrillation: a randomised non-inferiority trial. Lancet 2009;374(9689):534–42.

24. Maisel WH. Left atrial appendage occlusion–closure or just the beginning? N Engl J Med 2009;360(25): 2601–3.

25. FDA. FDA executive summary: Boston Scientific WATCHMAN left atrial appendage closure therapy. Prepared for the December 11, 2013 meeting of the Circulatory System Devices Panel. 2013. Available at: http://www.fda.gov/downloads/AdvisoryCommittees/CommitteesMeetingMaterials/MedicalDevices/MedicalDevicesAdvisoryCommittee/CirculatorySystemDevicesPanel/UCM377356.pdf. Accessed January 21, 2014.

26. Reddy VY, Holmes D, Doshi SK, et al. Safety of percutaneous left atrial appendage closure: results from the Watchman Left Atrial Appendage System for Embolic Protection in Patients with AF (PROTECT AF) clinical trial and the Continued Access Registry. Circulation 2011;123(4):417–24.

27. Kar S, Doshi S, Swarup V, et al. Long term efficacy of left atrial appendage closure with WATCHMAN device. Eur Heart J 2013;34(Suppl 1).

28. Dewilde WJ, Oirbans T, Verheugt FW, et al. Use of clopidogrel with or without aspirin in patients taking oral anticoagulant therapy and undergoing percutaneous coronary intervention: an open-label, randomised, controlled trial. Lancet 2013;381(9872): 1107–15.

29. FDA. Brief summary of the Circulatory System Devices panel meeting – December 11, 2013. 2013. Available at: http://www.fda.gov/downloads/AdvisoryCommittees/CommitteesMeetingMaterials/MedicalDevices/MedicalDevicesAdvisoryCommittee/CirculatorySystemDevicesPanel/UCM378634.pdf. Accessed January 21, 2014.

30. Reddy VY, Doshi SK, Sievert H, et al. Percutaneous left atrial appendage closure for stroke prophylaxis in patients with atrial fibrillation: 2.3-year follow-up of the PROTECT AF (Watchman Left Atrial Appendage System for Embolic Protection in Patients with Atrial Fibrillation) trial. Circulation 2013; 127(6):720–9.

31. Viles-Gonzalez JF, Kar S, Douglas P, et al. The clinical impact of incomplete left atrial appendage closure with the Watchman device in patients with atrial fibrillation: a PROTECT AF (Percutaneous Closure of the Left Atrial Appendage Versus Warfarin Therapy for Prevention of Stroke in Patients With Atrial Fibrillation) substudy. J Am Coll Cardiol 2012;59(10):923–9.

32. Cooper NJ, Sutton AJ, Lu G, et al. Mixed comparison of stroke prevention treatments in individuals with nonrheumatic atrial fibrillation. Arch Intern Med 2006;166(12):1269–75.

33. Camm AJ, Lip GY, De Caterina R, et al. 2012 focused update of the ESC guidelines for the management of atrial fibrillation: an update of the 2010 ESC guidelines for the management of atrial fibrillation–developed with the special contribution of the European Heart Rhythm Association. Europace 2012;14(10):1385–413.

34. Alli O, Doshi S, Kar S, et al. Quality of life assessment in the randomized PROTECT AF (Percutaneous Closure of the Left Atrial Appendage Versus Warfarin Therapy for Prevention of Stroke in Patients With Atrial Fibrillation) trial of patients at risk for stroke with nonvalvular atrial fibrillation. J Am Coll Cardiol 2013;61(17):1790–8.

35. Reddy VY, Mobius-Winkler S, Miller MA, et al. Left atrial appendage closure with the Watchman device in patients with a contraindication for oral anticoagulation: the ASAP study (ASA Plavix Feasibility Study With Watchman Left Atrial Appendage Closure Technology). J Am Coll Cardiol 2013;61(25):2551–6.

36. Massarenti L, Yilmaz A. Incomplete endothelialization of left atrial appendage occlusion device 10 months after implantation. J Cardiovasc Electrophysiol 2012;23(12):1384–5.

37. Plicht B, Konorza TF, Kahlert P, et al. Risk factors for thrombus formation on the Amplatzer Cardiac Plug after left atrial appendage occlusion. JACC Cardiovasc Interv 2013;6(6):606–13.

38. Eikelboom JW, Connolly SJ, Brueckmann M, et al. Dabigatran versus warfarin in patients with mechanical heart valves. N Engl J Med 2013; 369(13):1206–14.

39. Park JW, Bethencourt A, Sievert H, et al. Left atrial appendage closure with Amplatzer cardiac plug in atrial fibrillation: initial European experience. Catheter Cardiovasc Interv 2011;77(5):700–6.

40. Lam YY. A new left atrial appendage occluder (Lifetech LAmbre device) for stroke prevention in atrial fibrillation. Cardiovasc Revasc Med 2013;14(3): 134–6.

Catheter-based Epicardial Closure of the Left Atrial Appendage

Francesco Santoro, MD[a], Luigi Di Biase, MD, PhD[a,b,c,d,*],
Pasquale Santangeli, MD[a,b], Rong Bai, MD[b],
Stephan Danik, MD[e], Conor Barrett, MD[e],
Rodney Horton, MD[b], J. David Burkhardt, MD[b],
Andrea Natale, MD[b,d,f,g,h,i]

KEYWORDS

- Endo-epicardial closure device • Epicardial closure device • Left atrial appendage
- Stroke prevention

KEY POINTS

- The left atrial appendage (LAA) is a trabeculated, tubular structure, in direct continuity with the left atrial cavity. Its anatomy could predispose to in situ thrombus formation, especially in patients with atrial fibrillation.
- Different technologies have been developed for LAA closure, including surgical and percutaneous techniques. Both types have shown several limits.
- A novel technique based on an endo-epicardial approach, the LARIAT system (SentreHeart, Palo Alto, CA, USA), recently has become available. It consists of snaring the LAA with an epicardial device, correctly positioned through connection of the epicardial and endocardial magnet-tipped guidewires.
- Little clinical data are present in the literature about this new approach. Some additional considerations are reported based on our early clinical experience.

INTRODUCTION

Atrial fibrillation (AF) is the most common cardiac arrhythmia,[1] affecting an estimated 6 million individuals in the United States.[1] Because AF mainly affects elderly people, its prevalence is expected to increase in parallel with the increasing age of the population, with a predicted 15.9 million cases by 2050.[2]

Stroke, the most serious complication of AF, occurs in 5% of non-anticoagulated patients every year. The risk of stroke increases substantially with age, from 1.5% in individuals aged 50 to 59 years to 23.5% for those aged 80 to 89 years.[3] In

The authors have nothing to disclose.

[a] Department of Cardiology, University of Foggia, viale pinto 1, Foggia 71100, Italy; [b] Department of Cardiology, Texas Cardiac Arrhythmia Institute, St. David's Medical Center, 1015 East 32nd street, Suite 408, Austin, TX 78705, USA; [c] Division of Cardiology, Montefiore Hospital, Albert Einstein College of Medicine, 111 East 210th Street, Bronx, NY 10467, USA; [d] Department of Biomedical Engineering, University of Texas, 107 W. Dean Keeton, BME Building, Austin, TX 78712, USA; [e] Department of Cardiology, Al-Sabah Arrhythmia Institute (AI), St. Luke's Hospital, 1111 Amsterdam Ave, New York, NY 10025, USA; [f] EP Services, California Pacific Medical Center, 2100 Webster Street, San Francisco, CA 94115, USA; [g] Division of Cardiology, Stanford University, 300 Pasteur Drive, Palo Alto, CA 94305, USA; [h] Division of Cardiovascular Medicine, Case Western Reserve University, University Hospitals of Cleveland, 11100 Euclid Avenue, Cleveland, OH 44106-5038, USA; [i] Interventional Electrophysiology, Department of Cardiology, Scripps Clinic, 10666 N Torrey Pines Rd, La Jolla, CA 92037, USA
* Corresponding author. 1015 East 32nd Street, Suite 408, Austin, TX 78705.
E-mail address: dibbia@gmail.com

Intervent Cardiol Clin 3 (2014) 219–227
http://dx.doi.org/10.1016/j.iccl.2014.01.003
2211-7458/14/$ – see front matter © 2014 Elsevier Inc. All rights reserved.

addition, AF-associated strokes have the worst outcomes.[4]

Stroke is the third most frequent cause of death in the United States and the leading cause of serious disability. Therefore, stroke prophylaxis is a crucial component of management of AF. Although antiarrhythmic drugs and catheter ablation provide symptomatic relief for patients with AF, neither method is sufficiently reliable in preventing thromboembolic events, and long-term oral anticoagulation therapy is recommended ,irrespective of the rhythm management strategy.[5] Furthermore, data from Stroke Prevention in Nonrheumatic Atrial Fibrillation suggest that 15% of patients with AF suffer silent cerebral infarcts, the implications of which are not known.[6]

Stroke prevention in patients with AF has largely been based on the use of anticoagulation with warfarin, which reduces the risk of stroke by 60%,[7] and in some more recent patients stroke prevention has been based on the use of novel anticoagulants, such as the direct thrombin inhibitor, dabigatran.[8] Therapy with warfarin or the novel oral anticoagulants (eg, dabigatran or the selective factor Xa inhibitors apixaban and rivaroxaban) comes with a significant lifetime risk of major bleeding ranging from 1.4% to 3% per year in clinical trials,[9–11] which have excluded patients with a high risk of bleeding.

The cumulative incidence of major hemorrhage for patients 80 years of age or older has been estimated to be as high as 13.1 per 100 person-years, and these patients are not often enrolled in randomized clinical trials.[12] A significant proportion of patients with AF, ranging from 30% to 50%, does not receive anticoagulation because of relative or absolute contraindications or because of patient- and/or physician-pertinent barriers limiting the use of anticoagulation in clinical practice, including the perceived risk or fear of treatment-induced bleedings.[13]

For these reasons, different therapeutic approaches are currently being developed for stroke prevention in nonvalvular AF and potentially offer an alternative to anticoagulation therapy.

EPICARDIAL APPROACH

This recent strategy combines endocardial and epicardial approaches or uses an epicardial approach only. The endo-epicardial procedure requires 4 basic steps:

1. Pericardial and transseptal access.
2. Placement of 2 magnet-tipped guidewires, the first at the endocardial surface of the left atrial appendage (LAA) apex, via a femoral venous access and transseptal puncture. The second

is percutaneously introduced into the pericardium overlying the LAA apex.
3. Connection of the epicardial and endocardial magnet-tipped guidewires for stabilization of the LAA.
4. Snare capture of the LAA with closure confirmation and release of the pretied suture for LAA ligation. The main components of this system are illustrated in **Fig. 1**.

Pericardial access is obtained through a transthoracic puncture, done after proper asepsis of the subxiphoid area. Epicardial puncture is performed with the goal of achieving access only to the anterior surface of the heart to obtain the proper orientation to deliver the snare over the LAA. An inferior epicardial access is never recommended and in the case of an accidental inferior epicardial access it is advisable to re-access the epicardium rather than reposition the snare via the inferior orientation. A 17-G epidural needle is used for this procedure. The needle is introduced at a 45° angle toward the left scapula. Guided by fluoroscopy through anterior-posterior and lateral views, the operator gently advances the needle until it is close to the cardiac silhouette, where a light negative pressure is felt. The needle angle is adjusted according to the region the operator wishes to evaluate. This region is most frequently the medial third of the right ventricle, where no major coronary vessels can be found. To demonstrate the site of the needle tip precisely, 2 mL of contrast is injected as the needle approaches the heart silhouette. If the needle is outside the pericardial space, contrast media accumulate in the mediastinum. However, when the needle tip is inside the pericardial space, the contrast outlines the cardiac silhouette. This thin layer of contrast in the pericardial space confirms that the needle is correctly positioned. A lateral radiograph view, showing the anterior and posterior contours of the heart, represents the best view to ensure correct needle position. Indeed, through this view, anterior access can be confirmed and needle direction is clearly shown.

Finally, a 0.35-inch guidewire is introduced in the pericardial space through the puncture needle. The guidewire is also monitored with fluoroscopy and left in the pericardial space while the transseptal catheterization is performed.

Once the transseptal catheterization is completed, an 8.5-F SL1 catheter is directed anteriorly in the left atrium toward the LAA. To delineate the ostium and body of the LAA, a left atriagram is performed (**Fig. 2**). The 15-mm occlusion balloon catheter is back-loaded with a magnet-tipped 0.025-inch endocardial guidewire and inserted into the end of the SL1 transseptal catheter. The

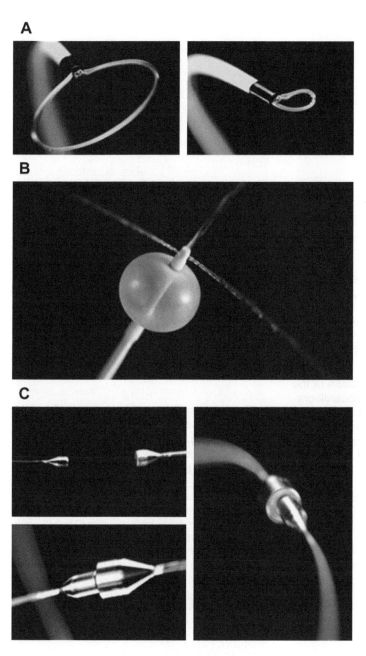

Fig. 1. Components of the endo-epicardial closure device. (*A*) LARIAT system suture device. (*B*) EndoCATH large occlusion balloon. (*C*) FindrWIRZ magnetic guide wire system. (*Courtesy of* SentreHeart, Palo Alto, CA.)

endocardial magnet-tipped guidewire is advanced to the apex of the LAA under fluoroscopic guidance. In clinical practice to advance the SL1 in the LAA, some operators use a pigtail catheter. To navigate the endocardial guidewire, a mild bend is placed at the end of the guidewire to allow steerability of the endocardial guidewire. The balloon catheter is then advanced over the wire into the LAA. Through the lumen of the balloon catheter an LAA angiogram (appendagram) is performed to evaluate the endocardial guidewire position, with a distal anterior LAA position being the favored location.

The epicardial access site is then sequentially dilated over the guidewire for placement of the 14-F soft-tipped epicardial guide cannula. The 0.035-inch epicardial magnet-tipped guidewire is placed through the epicardial sheath to achieve an end-to-end magnetic union with the endocardial guidewire. The attached magnet-tipped guidewires act as a controlled pathway for the delivery of the snare to the base of the LAA without the need for traction or grasping of the delicate LAA tissue (**Fig. 3**). Once the suture delivery device is positioned over the LAA, the endoCATH balloon

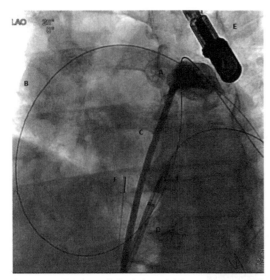

Fig. 2. Angiogram of the left atrial appendage (LAA), with assessment of the ostium position, LAA orientation, and LAA apex. A, LAA; B, epicardial wire; C, transseptal sheath; D, epicardial sheath; E, transesophageal probe; F, intracardial echocardiographic probe.

is used to position the snare at the ostium of the LAA (**Fig. 4**). 2D transesophageal echocardiography (TEE) is used to verify the anatomic position of the endoCATH balloon at the ostium of the LAA.

After confirmation of the balloon catheter at the LAA ostium, the snare is closed. A left atriagram is

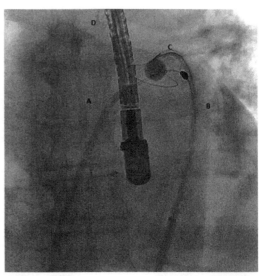

Fig. 4. EndoCATH balloon inflated in the LAA, facilitating the positioning of the LARIAT device (SentreHeart, Palo Alto, CA, USA) and the following snare. A, endocardial sheath with endoWire and EndoCath balloon inflated; B, epicardial sheath with epiWIRE and its magnet tip; C, LARIAT suture delivery device; D, transesophageal probe.

performed to confirm complete capture of the LAA and rule out the existence of a remnant trabeculated LAA (**Fig. 5**). After verifying LAA capture, the preloaded suture is released from the snare and tightened to exclude the LAA. Tightening is

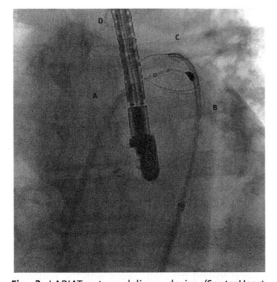

Fig. 3. LARIAT suture delivery device (SentreHeart, Palo Alto, CA, USA) positioned over the LAA, guided by the end-to-end union of endocardial and epicardial magnetic tips. A, endocardial sheath with endoWire and magnet tip; B, epicardial sheath with epiWIRE and its magnet tip; C, LARIAT suture delivery device; D, transesophageal probe.

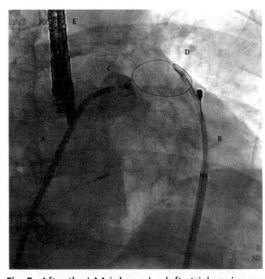

Fig. 5. After the LAA is bound, a left atrial angiogram is performed to verify its exclusion. A, endocardial sheath; B, epicardial sheath with epiWIRE and its magnet tip; C, exclusion of LAA appendage; D, LARIAT suture delivery device (SentreHeart, Palo Alto, CA, USA); E, transesophageal probe.

completed using a suture-tightening device that eliminates operator variability during tightening.

The snare is removed from the pericardial space. The suture is cut near the LAA with a suture cutter that passes over the suture. A pigtail catheter is placed in the pericardial space at least overnight. The epicardial catheter is attached to low suction to assess for any periprocedural pericardial effusions. A transthoracic echocardiogram is performed to rule out a pericardial effusion before the pericardial catheter is removed and is repeated 1 hour after the removal and at discharge. Intracardiac echocardiography can be considered both to deploy the system and to monitor for complications during the procedure.

Imaging During Procedure

A screening cardiac computed tomography (CT) scan is required for all patients, so that the morphology and the correct position of the LAA are appreciated by the physician. During the procedure, a left atriogram and 2D TEE are performed.

The 2D TEE is used to verify the anatomic position of the endocardial balloon at the ostium of the LAA, the eventual presence of a jet at the Doppler color flow after the suture is deployed, and the absence of pericardial effusion at the end of procedure.

One case reported the use of 3D TEE,[14] which could optimize

1. The assessment of the shape and size of the mouth of the LAA
2. The visualization of the epicardial catheter and by sequential cropping confirmed its location outside the LAA (this cannot be performed by 2D TEE)
3. A better assessment of the volume of the pericardial effusion developing or increasing during and/or after the procedure.

A limitation of 3D TEE as compared with 2D TEE is its lower resolution. In addition, cropping of the data sets is time-consuming and not instantaneous.

Inclusion Criteria

Inclusion criteria comprise the following:

a. Age 18 years or older
b. Nonvalvular AF
c. At least 1 risk factor for embolic stroke (CHADS≥1)
d. A poor candidate or ineligible for warfarin therapy (eg, labile international normalized ratio level, noncompliant, contraindicated) and/or a

warfarin failure (ie, transient ischemic attack or stroke while on warfarin therapy)
e. A life expectancy of at least 1 year

Exclusion Criteria

Exclusion criteria are as follows:

a. History of pericarditis
b. History of cardiac surgery
c. Pectus excavatum
d. Recent myocardial infarction within 3 months
e. Prior embolic event within the last 30 days
f. New York Heart Association functional class IV heart failure symptoms
g. Left ventricular function less than or equal to 30%
h. History of thoracic radiation.

These patients underwent a screening contrast cardiac CT scan. Additional exclusion criteria based on LAA anatomy included

1. A LAA width greater than or equal to 40 mm
2. A superiorly oriented LAA with the LAA apex directed behind the pulmonary trunk
3. Bilobed LAA or multilobed LAA in which lobes were oriented in different planes exceeding 40 mm
4. A posteriorly rotated heart

The incidence of patients who cannot be enrolled for this technique has been evaluated only in a large case series by Bartus and colleagues.[15] In this article, 16 (13.4%) patients were excluded after CT scan study, due to LAA size (8 [6.7%] patients with LAA width ≥40 mm) and unsuitable LAA orientation (8 [6.7%] patients).

Preliminary Studies and Results

The first study to demonstrate the feasibility and safety of the catheter-based epicardial LAA ligation device for the exclusion of the LAA was an animal model.[16] The study was performed on 26 dogs. After the intervention, a median sternotomy was realized acutely on 16 animals and no trauma or bleeding of the LAA on the epicardial surface was observed. Excision of the distal apex of the LAA was performed in all animals without showing any residual flow or incomplete exclusion. Endocardial examination showed complete closure at the origin of the atrial appendage except for 2 over 16 animals who had a diverticulum of less than or equal to 3 mm. Assessment of LAA exclusion was performed at 7 days, 1 month, and 3 months after the ligation procedure. Left atrial angiogram and intracardiac echocardiography imaging revealed 1 animal with a diverticulum of less than or equal to 3 mm at the 7 days' assessment, and complete LAA exclusion in all animals at 1 month. No trauma was observed at the LAA or epicardial surface in either the 7-day or the 1-month animals. Histologic examination at 7 days revealed endothelialization at the closure site with no necrosis or inflammatory response, and the examination at 1 month revealed complete endothelialized orifices of the LAA. At 3 months macroscopic examination showed an LAA almost completely incorporated into the visceral pericardium and histologic examination was similar to the 1-month follow-up.

Another study was performed on 9 dogs that were randomized to concomitant use of a transseptally placed endoluminal balloon within the LAA or not.[17] In all animals, LAA closure was complete without a leak. When the endoluminal balloon was used, there were no proximal residual LAA remnants in 5 of 5 (100%) animals; on the other hand, a proximal residual LAA remnant was present when the balloon-tipped catheter was not inflated during the procedure (3 of 4 animals without balloon inflation).

The first study to show feasibility of epicardial LAA ligation with the endo-epicardial approach in humans was done by Bartus and colleagues.[18] Thirteen patients were enrolled in the study, undergoing either concomitant mitral valve replacement (n = 2) or radiofrequency catheter ablation for AF (n = 11). Open-chest ligation of the LAA after mitral valve replacement was feasible and all patients had a complete closure. The intent to ligate the LAA during concomitant RF ablation for AF was completed in 10 of 11 patients. Nine of 10 patients had a complete LAA closure and one had a 1-mm jet identified by color flow Doppler. A small hemopericardium (≤50 mL) was noted after the procedure. At 60-day follow-up, 2 patients had a less than 2-mm opening by color flow Doppler detected by TEE.

A larger cohort of patients (n = 89) and a longer follow-up (1 year) in a study by Bartus and colleagues[15] gave more information about the efficacy and all possible complications of this technique. Immediate LAA closure was achieved in 85 of 89 patients attempted. Different conditions were related to unsuccessful ligation. Two patients had pericardial access–related complications: a right ventricular puncture, requiring drainage and observation, and a laceration of a superficial epigastric vessel, requiring cauterization to stop the bleeding. One patient had pericardial adhesions in the LAA sulcus. Another patient had his procedure aborted because of the inability to perform a transseptal puncture. A complication that did not compromise LAA epicardial closure occurred during the transseptal catheterization, resulting in perforation and hemopericardium successfully drained, because epicardial access was in place. A common symptom following the procedure was chest pain; 20 of 85 patients had it, and 2 of them developed pericarditis.

Complete closure was defined as a less than or equal to 1-mm jet by color flow Doppler. TEE performed 1 day, 30 days, and 90 days after the procedure revealed complete closure in 95% of patients in whom LAA ligation was attempted. In 1 patient, color Doppler echocardiography increased from less than or equal to 1-mm to a less than or equal to 2-mm color Doppler jet, but remained stable at 1-month and 3-month follow-up. No patients had a greater than or equal to 3-mm jet by color Doppler at 3 months, 1 had a less than or equal to 3-mm jet, and 2 had a less than or equal to 2-mm jet. Complete closure of the LAA was seen in 98% of patients undergoing 1-year follow-up TEE, and only one patient had a less than or equal to 2-mm color Doppler leak. At 1-year clinical follow-up there were 4 deaths: 2 patients died of sudden death, 1 had a hemorrhagic stroke secondary to an aneurysm, and another one had a lacunar stroke related to a hypertensive crisis.

A case series of 20 patients by Massumi and colleagues[19] showed that the exclusion of the LAA was successful in all patients. At the Doppler color flow of the LAA, only 1 patient had 1-mm jet. All of these results were confirmed with a 1-year TEE. There were 2 intraoperative complications: a perforation of the right ventricle with tamponade treated with emergent surgical exploration and repair, a pericardial effusion with tamponade physiology requiring pericardiocentesis. Three patients were rehospitalized for pericarditis less than 1 month after the procedure. One of these 3 patients also had moderate pericardial effusion treated with pericardial drainage, and the other 2 patients were treated conservatively. At 1-year clinical follow-up, no new strokes or cerebrovascular events were reported and only one patient died 50 days after the procedure from multiple organ failure.

ADDITIONAL CONSIDERATIONS

In the authors' early clinical experience a few issues appeared underreported in previous series. These issues include

1. Late serous pericardial effusion, which affects nearly one-third of patients; therefore, in clinical practice pericardial drainage is left in place for 2 to 3 days.

2. Thrombus formation between the procedure and 1-month follow-up is possible. Therefore, it could be safer not to stop oral anticoagulant therapy after the procedure if the patient does not have a contraindication. The anticoagulation management in these patients is still under investigation. A case of early LARIAT reopening has been reported by the authors' group.[20]

Epicardial Approach

The overall complication rate for such an approach is relatively low in experienced centers with reported rates of 4% to 7%.[21] Pericardial bleeding because of right ventricular puncture remains the most common complication. In addition, the risk of ventricular pseudoaneurysm, ventricular hematoma, and coronary venous or coronary artery laceration exists. Furthermore, damage to surrounding thoracic and abdominal structures has been reported, even in experienced centers, including abdominal vessel bleeding and hepatic hematoma.[22]

Pericarditis and Pericardial Effusion

Pericarditis and pericardial effusion reflects probably the most common complication. In the authors' clinical practice it affects nearly one-third of patients, with an incidence of 30%. Pericarditis occurs in virtually all patients to some extent as the result of a local inflammatory response. The clinical manifestation varies from mild pericarditis to large serous pericardial effusion and, rarely, cardiac tamponade. Late serous pericardial effusion is not an uncommon finding as a result of a chronic inflammation process. Therefore, the pericardial drainage is left in place for at least 2 to 3 days. As a matter of fact, chest pain, a frequent symptom after the procedure, could also be related to mild pericarditis.

Thrombus Formation in Patients Taken Off Blood Thinner

Thrombus formation between the procedure and 1-month follow-up has been observed. Therefore, because of leak, LARIAT reopening, and thrombus formation, anticoagulation discontinuation should be decided after 1-month follow-up TEE unless totally contraindicated.

Incomplete Closure of LAA

The rate of this phenomenon is not well defined. Indeed, only Bartus and colleagues[18] and Massumi and colleagues[19] described some cases in their series, with a small cohort of patients. Suture reopening has been reported in both patients with optimal acute results and patients with less than or equal to 2-mm leak and has been observed at both 1 month and a later follow-up (**Fig. 6**). The authors' registry showed that 27% of patients have various degrees of LAA leak after the LARIAT procedure. Most of these leaks can be successfully closed with smaller closure devices.

Laceration of the LAA

This complication has been observed only in a few patients.[23] Although this complication is rare, it is potentially lethal and all physicians should be aware of it.

Effect on Arrhythmia Burden

Complete ligation and elimination of LAA could have a positive benefit in atrial arrhythmia burden reduction. In a case series of 18 patients, Lakkireddy and colleagues[24] reported a 34% reduction of atrial arrhythmia burden at 3 months after ligation. Furthermore, in 11% patients, AF completely disappeared. The relevance of the effect of LAA ligation on the atrial arrhythmia burden requires further investigation.

NEW PERCUTANEOUS NONSURGICAL TECHNIQUES
AEGIS

AEGIS is an electrocardiogram-guided LAA capture and ligation system that requires the epicardial approach only. It has been tested in animals[25,26] and recently in about 50 patients. It permits LAA closure in the closed pericardial space with a single sheath puncture with 2 components: an appendage grasper and a ligator. The

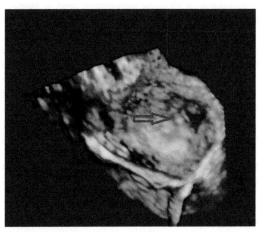

Fig. 6. 3D TEE shows incomplete closure of LAA at 1-month follow-up after LARIAT (SentreHeart, Palo Alto, CA, USA) implantation. The red arrow indicates the opening of the LAA.

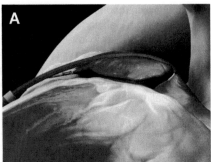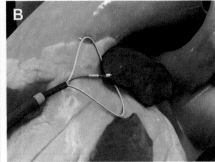

Fig. 7. (*A*, *B*) AEGIS electrocardiogram-guided LAA capture and ligation system. (*Courtesy of* Aegis Medical Innovations Inc., Vancouver, BC, Canada.)

grasper has an articulating jaw with specially mounted electrodes that make the identification of the position and tissue capture possible by means of electrical signals (**Fig. 7**). Between the 2 jaws an atrial electrogram is recorded and identifies the tissue captured. Recordings between each jaw and the shaft, and bipolar recordings along the shaft, permit identification of the grasper's position relative to electrically active cardiac tissue. Once the system is positioned near the LAA, the LAA is controlled by the grasper and a hollow suture loop is advanced over the grasper, around the free margin of the appendage, and to its base. Once the loop is in position, it is cinched down, occluding the LAA, after which the wire is removed, leaving only the suture behind.

EPITEK

EPITEK is a fiberoptic endoscope that allows visualization of the pericardial space and of the LAA. The device includes a tool used to grasp the appendage, a closure apparatus, and a system to deploy, control, and position the closure tool. The LAA grasper has 2 nontraumatic metal jaws, one lumen for a pretied suture and the other lumen for a shape-set nitinol wire. The Anchorage scope has a 75°field of view and a standard endoscope connection. Preclinical testing was conducted from December 2006 to February 2008 on animals (porcine, canine). In the early human testing access was achieved in 78% of cases and a good device position was achieved in only 41%. Therefore optimizing the device function and handling is still necessary.

SUMMARY

This novel approach provides new perspectives to those patients with AF that cannot use anticoagulation therapy. However, the role of this technique has to be validated in large and prospective registries.

REFERENCES

1. Wolf PA, Abbott RD, Kannel WB. Atrial fibrillation as an independent risk factor for stroke: the Framingham Study. Stroke 1991;22:983–8.
2. Lloyd-Jones DM, Wang TJ, Leip EP, et al. Lifetime risk for development of atrial fibrillation: the Framingham Heart Study. Circulation 2004;110:1042–6.
3. Lin HJ, Wolf PA, Kelly-Hayes M, et al. Stroke severity in atrial fibrillation. The Framingham Study. Stroke 1996;27:1760–4.
4. Whitlock RP, Healey JS, Connolly SJ. Left atrial appendage occlusion does not eliminate the need for warfarin. Circulation 2009;120:1927–32.
5. Sherman DG. Stroke prevention in atrial fibrillation pharmacologic rate versus rhythm control. Stroke 2007;38:615–7.
6. Stewart S, Hart CL, Hole DJ, et al. Population prevalence, incidence, and predictors of atrial fibrillation in the Renfrew/Paisley study. Heart 2001;86:516–21.
7. Hart RG, Pearce LA, Aguilar MI. Meta-analysis: antithrombotic therapy to prevent stroke in patients who have nonvalvular atrial fibrillation. Ann Intern Med 2007;146:857–67.
8. Connolly SJ, Ezekowitz MD, Yusuf S, et al. Dabigatran versus warfarin in patients with atrial fibrillation. N Engl J Med 2009;361:1139–51.
9. Connolly SJ, Eikelboom J, Joyner C, et al. Apixaban in patients with atrial fibrillation. N Engl J Med 2011; 364:806–17.
10. Cleland JG, Coletta AP, Buga L, et al. Clinical trials update from the American Heart Association Meeting 2010: EMPHASIS-HF, RAFT, TIM-HF, Tele-HF, ASCEND-HF, ROCKET-AF, and PROTECT. Eur J Heart Fail 2011;13:460–5.
11. Eikelboom JW, Wallentin L, Connolly SJ, et al. Risk of bleeding with 2 doses of dabigatran compared with warfarin in older and younger patients with atrial

fibrillation: an analysis of the randomized evaluation of long-term anticoagulant therapy (RE-LY) trial. Circulation 2011;123:2363–72.

12. Hylek EM, Evans-Molina C, Shea C, et al. Major hemorrhage and tolerability of warfarin in the first year of therapy among elderly patients with atrial fibrillation. Circulation 2007;115:2689–96.

13. Bungard TJ, Ghali WA, Teo KK, et al. Why do patients with atrial fibrillation not receive warfarin? Arch Intern Med 2000;160:41–6.

14. Joshi D, Mazimba S, Neal Kay G, et al. Role of live/real time three-dimensional transesophageal echocardiography in the percutaneous epicardial closure of the left atrial appendage. Echocardiography 2012. http://dx.doi.org/10.1111/j.1540-8175.2012.01821.x.

15. Bartus K, Han FT, Bednarek J, et al. Percutaneous left atrial appendage suture ligation using the LARIAT device in patients with atrial fibrillation: initial clinical experience. J Am Coll Cardiol 2013;62(2):108–18.

16. Lee RJ, Bartus K, Yakubov SJ. Catheter-based left atrial appendage (LAA) ligation for the prevention of embolic events arising from the LAA: initial experience in a canine model. Circ Cardiovasc Interv 2010;3(3):224–9.

17. Singh SM, Dukkipati SR, d'Avila A, et al. Percutaneous left atrial appendage closure with an epicardial suture ligation approach: a prospective randomized pre-clinical feasibility study. Heart Rhythm 2010;7(3):370–6.

18. Bartus K, Bednarek J, Myc J, et al. Feasibility of closed-chest ligation of the left atrial appendage in humans. Heart Rhythm 2011;8(2):188–93.

19. Massumi A, Chelu MG, Nazeri A, et al. Initial experience with a novel percutaneous left atrial appendage exclusion device in patients with atrial fibrillation, increased stroke risk, and contraindications to anticoagulation. Am J Cardiol 2013;111(6):869–73.

20. Di Biase L, Burkhardt JD, Gibson DN, et al. 2D and 3D TEE evaluation of an early reopening of the LARIAT epicardial left atrial appendage closure device. Heart Rhythm 2013. http://dx.doi.org/10.1016/j.hrthm.2013.08.023. pii:S1547-5271(13)00898-9.

21. Della Bella P, Brugada J, Zeppenfeld K, et al. Epicardial ablation for ventricular tachycardia: a European multicenter study. Circ Arrhythm Electrophysiol 2011;4(5):653–9.

22. Koruth JS, Aryana A, Dukkipati SR, et al. Unusual complications of percutaneous epicardial access and epicardial mapping and ablation of cardiac arrhythmias. Circ Arrhythm Electrophysiol 2011;4(6):882–8.

23. Keating VP, Kolibash CP, Khandheria BK, et al. Left atrial laceration with epicardial ligation device. Ann Thorac Cardiovasc Surg 2013. [Epub ahead of print].

24. Lakkireddy DR, Earnest M, Janga P, et al. Effect of endoepicardial percutaneous left atrial appendage ligation (Lariat) on arrhythmia burden in patients with atrial fibrillation. J Am Coll Cardiol 2013;61(10):E385.

25. Friedman PA, Asirvatham SJ, Dalegrave C, et al. Percutaneous epicardial left atrial appendage closure: preliminary results of an electrogram guided approach. J Cardiovasc Electrophysiol 2009;20:908–15.

26. Bruce CJ, Stanton CM, Asirvatham SJ, et al. Percutaneous epicardial left atrial appendage closure: intermediate-term results. J Cardiovasc Electrophysiol 2011;22:64–70.

Managing the Left Atrial Appendage in the Era of Minimally Invasive Surgery

Alessandro Montecalvo, MD, Ralph J. Damiano Jr, MD*

KEYWORDS

- Atrial fibrillation • Left atrial appendage occlusion • Cox-Maze procedure

KEY POINTS

- Patient demand for minimally invasive techniques is expected to grow exponentially.
- We must continue to innovate and refine less invasive methods for left atrial appendage occlusion that focus on providing the superior results of the Cox-Maze procedure with endoscopic approaches that facilitate quicker patient recovery, faster healing, improved cosmetics, and overall lower patient morbidity.

 Videos of stapler resection of the left atrial appendage through the left thoracotomy and of the AtriClip Gillinov-Cosgrove atrial exclusion device accompany this article at http://www.interventional.theclinics.com/

INTRODUCTION

Atrial fibrillation (AF) is the most prevalent arrhythmia encountered in clinical practice with greater than 2.2 million people in the United States being affected.[1] Oral anticoagulant therapy (OAC), most commonly with warfarin, has been used to reduce risk of stroke in patients with nonvalvular AF who are at a high risk of thromboembolism (TE).[2] Unfortunately, warfarin is underused in these patients, mainly because of patient and health practitioner concerns and clinical data have suggested that only 50% to 60% of eligible patients are actually taking it.[3] Furthermore, clinical trials have demonstrated that a significant portion of patients on warfarin are not adequately anticoagulated, placing them at an increased risk of stroke.

Alternative treatment strategies to prevent TE have been tested in patients with AF. Because the left atrial appendage (LAA) has been well recognized as the principal source of embolism in nonvalvular heart disease and AF, it is not surprising that many of those efforts have been directed mostly toward the surgical management of LAA. In a review of operative, autopsy, and transesophageal echocardiographic (TEE) studies, Blackshear and Odell[4] identified the LAA as the source of left atrial thrombi in up to 90% of nonvalvular and 57% of valvular AF patients, respectively. Concurrently, minimally invasive cardiac surgery techniques have emerged to treat selected patients with AF, refractory to medical therapy, with surgical ablation and LAA resection through smaller, sternal-sparing incisions. The goals are to achieve sinus rhythm restoring, reduce incidence of TE, and achieve quicker recovery and an improved patient satisfaction with a more cosmetically appealing surgery.

This article examines the history of LAA occlusion and the efficacy of the various surgical techniques; it also provides a brief overview of

Dr Damiano receives consulting fees from AtriCure and Medtronic, and receives research funding from Edwards and AtriCure.

Division of Cardiothoracic Surgery, Barnes-Jewish Hospital, Washington University School of Medicine, 1 Barnes-Jewish Hospital Plaza, St Louis, MO 63110, USA

* Corresponding author. Division of Cardiothoracic Surgery, Barnes-Jewish Hospital, Washington University School of Medicine, Suite 3108 Queeny Tower, 1 Barnes-Jewish Hospital Plaza, St Louis, MO 63110.
E-mail address: damianor@wustl.edu

Intervent Cardiol Clin 3 (2014) 229–238
http://dx.doi.org/10.1016/j.iccl.2013.12.004
2211-7458/14/$ – see front matter © 2014 Elsevier Inc. All rights reserved.

the minimally invasive surgical strategy adopted at the authors' Center to manage the LAA.

LAA

The LAA is a long, tubular, hooked structure, usually crenellated, with a narrow junction with the venous component of the left atrium. In contrast, the right counterpart is more broad-based and triangular, forming a wide junction to the right atrium that makes blood stasis less likely (**Fig. 1**).[5] It originates from primordial atrial tissue, separate from the nascent pulmonary veins that subsequently are incorporated gradually. Clinical studies using TEE[6,7] and magnetic resonance angiography[8] demonstrate significant heterogeneity among patients in LAA size, wall thickness, and morphology (**Fig. 2**). The LAA is located on the lateral wall of the heart close to the circumflex artery, which is relevant for surgical occlusion. On the endocardial surface, it is within 1 cm of the mitral valve annulus and the orifice of the left superior pulmonary vein.

Histopathologic studies demonstrate that the LAA contains stretch receptors that mediate thirst, and its endocrine function, throughout the release

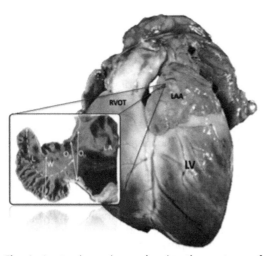

Fig. 1. Anatomic specimens showing the anatomy of the LAA. Notice the difference between the trabecular LAA and the smooth-walled left atrial cavity, which have diverse embryonic origins. L, length; LA, left atrium; LV, left ventricle; Oa, anatomic orifice; Oe, echocardiographic orifice; RVOT, right ventricle outflow tract; W, width. ([*Inset*] *Adapted from* Veinot JP, Harrity PJ, Gentile F, et al. Anatomy of the normal left atrial appendage: a quantitative study of age-related changes in 500 autopsy hearts: implications for echocardiographic examination. Circulation 1997;96:3112–15; and [*Remainder*] *From* Scanavacca MI, Venancio AC, Pisani CF, et al. Percutaneous transatrial access to the pericardial space for epicardial mapping and ablation. Circ Arrhythm Electrophysiol 2011;4:331–6.)

of the ANP, is responsible for the fluid homeostasis. The LAA is also recognized as the most distensible part of the left atrium, playing a role in the overall left heart mechanics.[9] An underappreciated role of the LAA is as a trigger for recurrent AF after catheter ablation, as was seen in 27% of patients in a recent large review of 987 cases.[10] This observation stresses the importance of achieving electrical isolation of the LAA while performing ablative procedures on AF patients.

HISTORY OF LAA OCCLUSION

Cerebral infarction is the most devastating complication of AF. The relationship between rheumatic mitral valve disease, systemic embolism, and the LAA was first noted in 1955 by Belcher and Somerville.[11] LAA obliteration itself was suggested as an adjunct to mitral valvotomy before the advent of cardiopulmonary bypass. The first clinical resection of the LAA, as a prophylaxis of recurrent arterial embolism, was performed by Madden in 1949.[12] The results of LAA obliteration in 8 patients involving ligation and appendectomy were later reviewed by Leonard and Cogan,[13] who noted a high complication rate, including 3 deaths, 1 paraplegia, and 3 peripheral emboli, and recommended that the procedure "should be abandoned." Since then, surgical closure of the LAA has been performed primarily in patients with concomitant mitral valve disease with different results. LAA occlusion surgery gained new light during the 1990s thanks to 2 different developments: the introduction of the Cox-Maze procedure to treat AF and the extensive use of intraoperative TEE study to assess the success or failure of the LAA closure techniques (**Fig. 3**).

The Maze procedure, introduced by James Cox in 1987, has always incorporated the excision of the LAA. In a series of almost 200 consecutive cases, the procedure demonstrated a very low stroke incidence at 5-year follow-up.[14] This high success rate has been attributed not only to eliminating atrial arrhythmias but also to the excision of the LAA (**Fig. 4**). A more recent study from the authors' group involved 450 patients, who were followed for a mean period of 6.9 years after a Cox-Maze procedure. The yearly rate of stroke in patients who discontinued all anticoagulants was 0.1% in patients with a CHADS$_2$ score of 0 or 1% and 0.3% in those with a CHADS$_2$ score ≥ 2 (**Table 1**).[15] Interestingly, the risk of stroke was not influenced by whether the patients were on OACs.

SURGICAL TECHNIQUES FOR LAA OCCLUSION

Johnson and colleagues[16] have described the LAA as "our most lethal attachment." In that

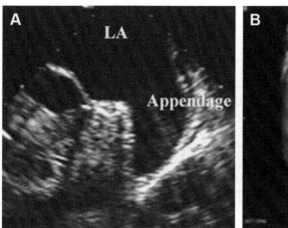
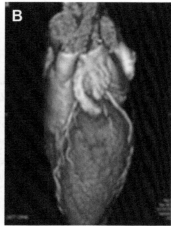

Fig. 2. Image techniques commonly used to study LAA morphology. (*A*) Echocardiographic study. (*B*) MR study. ([*A*] *From* E-chocardiography journal: an electronic journal of cardiac ultrasound. Available at: http://rwjms1. umdnj.edu/shindler/a_fib.html. Accessed December 16, 2013; and [*B*] Kerut EK. Anatomy of the left atrial appendage. Echocardiography 2008;25(6):669–73; with permission.)

report 437 patients were enrolled over a period of 3 years and received a prophylactic LAA excision. Twenty-one perioperative cerebrovascular accidents were reported, but no later strokes or TEE demonstrable thrombi were seen at follow-up. Consequently, the authors recommended an aggressive strategy of LAA excision in patients undergoing heart operations.

Currently, only a few centers and surgeons routinely close the LAA while performing cardiac surgery, and this despite that the European Society of Cardiology guidelines for the management of AF suggest that patients with contraindication to chronic OAC should be considered as candidates for LAA occlusion.[17] With regards to surgery, the American College of Cardiology/American Heart Association 2006 guidelines for management of patients with valvular heart

disease recommend patients undergo amputation of the LAA concomitantly to mitral valve surgery, to reduce the incidence of postoperative thromboembolic events.[18]

Unfortunately, the best surgical method to accomplish a successful LAA occlusion is still to be determined. Generally, the LAA has been approached from both epicardial and endocardial methods, which can be broadly divided into 2 categories: *exclusion* and *excision*. Within the first group are running or mattressed sutures, with or without felt pledgets, or, more recently, proprietary "cliplike" devices. On the other hand, the excision method includes a stapled excision or removal and oversew (**Fig. 5**). The excision technique confirms that removal of part of the appendage, however, can have a risk of hemorrhage and the potential for thrombus formation within the incompletely

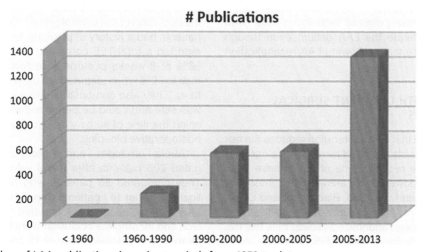

 # Publications

Fig. 3. Number of LAA publications in various periods from 1950 to date.

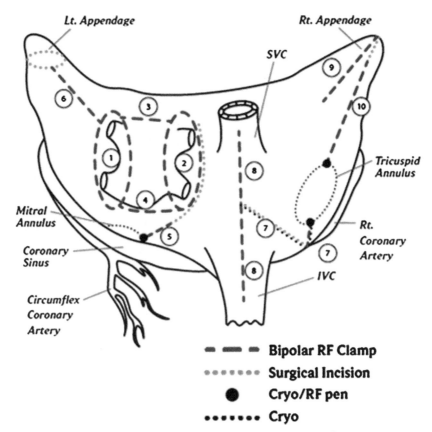

Fig. 4. Cox-Maze IV lesions' set as performed at the authors' institution. IVC, inferior vena cava; Lt. Appendage, left atrial appendage; RF, radiofrequency; Rt. Appendage, right atrial appendage; Rt. Coronary Artery, right coronary artery; SVC, superior vena cava. (*From* Lall SC, Melby SJ, Voeller RK, et al. The effect of ablation technology on surgical outcomes after the Cox-Maze procedure: a propensity analysis. J Thorac Cardiovasc Surg 2007;133:389–96; with permission.)

resected appendage with partial remaining stumps. Epicardial approaches are best suited toward bilateral thoracotomy access. Endocardial techniques can be used most commonly with a right mini-thoracotomy approach. Both purse-string and running closure techniques have been used to obliterate the LAA ostium even though they frequently fail by allowing LAA recanalization (**Fig. 6**).

RESULTS WITH DIFFERENT SURGICAL TECHNIQUES

The evidence that LAA obliteration reduces the risk of stroke consists mostly of retrospective case series and case reports, none of which have been adequately powered to answer this important question. As early as 1996, Blackshear and Odell[4] from the Mayo Clinic group advocated the need of a prospective, randomized clinical trial, but this was not performed until 2005. The Left Atrial Appendage Occlusion Study trial was the first randomized, single-center, placebo-controlled study of surgical LAA occlusion in patients with risk factors for AF and stroke undergoing concurrent coronary artery bypass grafting surgery.[19] Seventy-seven patients were randomized to either the occlusion or the control group, but only 32% of patients had a history of previous AF. The authors reported a total TEE-confirmed occlusion rate of 66% at 8-weeks postoperative follow-up, which rose to 72% when staples were used instead of sutures. They also demonstrated that LAA occlusion was safe and could be performed without lengthening the time of surgery or increasing the rate of postoperative bleeding.

Garcia-Fernandez and colleagues[20] investigated 205 patients after mitral valve operations. They compared 58 patients who had their LAA ligated against 147 patients who did not have their LAA ligated. The authors found that no LAA occlusion and incomplete occlusion were the major risk factors for the development of TE sequelae over a mean follow-up time of 69 months. In this series,

Table 1
CHADS$_2$ Score scale is used to formulate a clinical prediction of estimated stroke risk in patients with nonrheumatic atrial fibrillation, based on various risk factors

CHADS Risk Scoring System		
Risk Factor	Points	Stroke Rate (95% CI)[a]
Congestive heart failure	+1	Score of 0 1.9%
Hypertension	+1	Score of 1 2.8%
Age ≥75 y	+1	Score of 2 4.0%
Diabetes	+1	Score of 3 5.9%
Stroke/TIA	+2	Score of 4 8.5%
Maximum score 6		Score of 5 12.5%
		Score of 6 18.9

Abbreviations: CI, confidence interval; TIA, transient ischemic attack.
[a] Per 100 patients-year without antithrombotic therapy.
From Castellano JM, Chinitz J, Willner J, et al. Mechanisms of stroke in atrial fibrillation. Cardiac Electrophysiol Clin 2014;6: in press; with permission.

an incomplete LAA occlusion was more dangerous than no occlusion at all. Kanderian and co-workers[21] reviewed 137 of 2546 patients undergoing surgical LAA closure, who had TEE after surgery by any reason. Fifty-two patients (38%) had the excision, and 85 (62%) underwent exclusion (73 with suture and 12 with stapler) of the LAA. Although overall success closure was only 40%, the success rate was significantly different among groups: 73%, 23%, and 0% in excision,

suture exclusion, and stapler exclusion, respectively (*P*<.001). LAA thrombus was present in 41% of patients with unsuccessful LAA exclusion versus 0% in the entire excision group. The other interesting finding from both the Left Atrial Appendage Occlusion Study and Kanderian's report is the pattern of failure reported for each technique. The suture exclusion method had a tendency to fail because of persistent flow into the LAA, whereas the stapled exclusion group had a tendency to fail due to the presence of a remnant appendage defined as larger than 1 cm. The authors concluded that when surgical LAA closure is planned, excision of the appendage is the most reliable technique and anticoagulation should not be discontinued until successful closure is confirmed by follow-up TEE evaluation.

Unfortunately, excision of the left appendage is difficult, if not impossible, to achieve during minimally invasive mitral valve surgery that is usually performed via a right thoracotomy. Moreover, excision also requires cardiopulmonary bypass. Thus, these results suggest the need for the development of a more effective means of less invasive LAA exclusion strategy.

MINIMALLY INVASIVE APPROACHES

Management of the LAA in minimally invasive surgery varies mostly on the surgical approaches used, including bilateral mini-thoracotomy and right mini-thoracotomy. In right mini-thoracotomy approaches, commonly used in case of concomitant mitral valve surgery, LAA exclusion with purse-string or running sutures has been the most common modality used. However, concerns

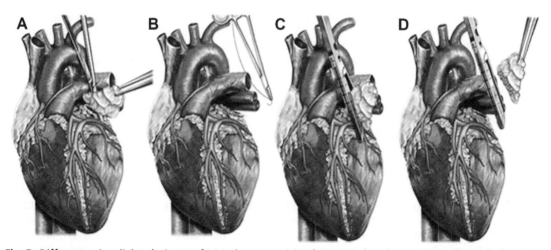

Fig. 5. Different epicardial techniques of LAA closure: excision by removal and oversew (*A, B*), stapled excision (*C, D*). (*Adapted from* Chatterjee S, Alexander JC, Pearson PJ, et al. Left atrial appendage occlusion: lessons learned from surgical and transcatheter experiences. Ann Thorac Surg 2011;92:2283–92; with permission.)

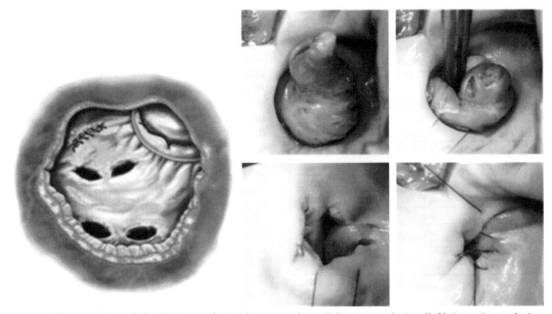

Fig. 6. Different endocardial techniques of LAA closure: endocardial suture exclusion (*left*), inversion technique (*right*). ([*Left*] *Adapted from* Chatterjee S, Alexander JC, Pearson PJ, et al. Left atrial appendage occlusion: lessons learned from surgical and transcatheter experiences. Ann Thorac Surg 2011;92:2283–92; with permission; and [*Right*] *Adapted from* Hernandez-Estefania R, Levy Praschker B, Bastarrika G, et al. Left atrial appendage occlusion by invagination and double suture technique. Eur J Cardiothorac Surg 2012;41(1):134–6; with permission.)

of high failure rate and early recanalization have tempered these techniques.[19] As a result, pericardial reinforced or inversion techniques, with the invagination of the LAA into the body of the left atrium, excision, and direct suturing, as was originally performed in the Cox-Maze procedure, are probably, in this scenario, the most efficacious method to achieve complete LAA occlusion.

Because the LAA can also be accessed from the pericardial space, several devices have been specifically designed to offer a minimally invasive solution for the LAA management. The Wolf procedure allows for stapler resection of the LAA through the left thoracotomy[22] (Video 1; available at: http://www.interventional.theclinics.com/). In 2003, Blackshear and colleagues[23] described successful thoracoscopic obliteration of the LAA using a stapled or snare technique. The procedure was completed in 14 of 15 patients, with one conversion to thoracotomy for bleeding. At a mean follow-up of 42 months, there were 2 strokes and 2 deaths, but TEE results were not reported. More recently, several cliplike LAA occlusion devices have been developed for the thoracoscopic approach[24] and tested on animal models, but at present only one device has gained the approval for clinical use in the United States and Europe: the AtriClip Gillinov-Cosgrove atrial exclusion device (AED; AtriCure Inc, West Chester, OH, USA) **(Fig. 7).**

First introduced in 2006, it has undergone several refinements and is currently a third-generation device. The AtriClip AED consists of 3 different components. The skeleton of the AED is composed of 2 parallel, straight, rigid titanium tubes with elastic nitinol springs arranged at a 90° angle at both ends of the tubes. The rigid titanium tubes are covered with a urethane elastomer, and the entire skeleton is covered with 2 knit-braided polyester sheaths, which promote rapid ingrowth of fibrous tissue. The device comes in 4 different sizes and a specifically designed long-armed delivery tool has been developed to facilitate the thoracoscopic application of the device. If the AED is deployed and the position on the LAA is judged to be suboptimal, the AED can be repositioned and reapplied by reattaching the delivery tool to the implanted AED. In fact, one of the principal disadvantages of other currently available epicardial occlusion devices is that they deliver a "permanent first implant" and are not able to be adjusted. When compared with those devices, the AED offers 2 advantages: (1) easy reapplication and (2) elimination of the risk of bleeding. These advantages enhance its safety when used on the beating heart, off cardiopulmonary bypass, particularly with a thoracoscopic approach. The deployment of the AED usually takes less than 10 seconds and the specific delivery tool makes it possible

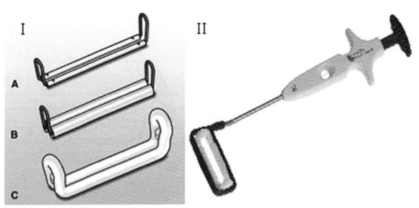

Fig. 7. (*I*) Components of the AED. (A) Titanium skeleton, (B) urethane elastomer, (C) knit-braided polyester sheaths. (*II*) Delivery tool. ([*I*] *From* Fumoto H, Gillinov AM, Ootaki Y, et al. A novel device for left atrial appendage exclusion: the third-generation atrial exclusion device. J Thorac Cardiovasc Surg 2008;136(4):1019–27; with permission; and [*II*] *Courtesy of* AtriCure Inc, Wests Chester, OH.)

to exploit the advantages of the AED, especially in minimally invasive surgery settings.

At the authors' institution, they have begun using this device via a thoracoscopic approach. Patients are intubated with a double lumen endotracheal tube and placed supine on the operating room table with the left chest wall elevated by 20° to 30°. Three ports are placed on the lateral chest wall. The pericardium is open below the phrenic nerve and the LAA is exposed. The application technique is demonstrated in Video 2 (available at: http://www.interventional.theclinics.com/).

The validity of the concept of the AED, along with its safety and efficacy, has been tested in canines[25] and primates.[26] These studies showed that the AtriClip AED was able to achieve a 100% successful occlusion rate in both early and mid-term follow-up, without interfering with surrounding structures (pulmonary artery, left atrium, left circumflex artery) or compromising any hemodynamic parameters (**Fig. 8**). Gross and histologic examination provided evidence of complete incorporation of the AED secondary to tissue ingrowth along the 2 polyester sheaths, which helped prevent device migration. In a cross-section of the occlusion site, the LAA walls beneath the AED were firmly adherent to each other, with a clear and smooth endocardial surface without any cul-de-sac formation. Ninety days after the implantation, the LAA was reduced to an atrophied remnant with an internal cavity fully occupied by a well-organized thrombus or dense connective tissue. Moreover, that remnant appeared to be electrically isolated from the remainder of the left atrium.[21]

In 2010, Salzberg and coworkers[27] presented preliminary data from the first human trial specifically designed to evaluate the safety and effectiveness of the AED in patients with AF who were undergoing cardiac surgery. Thirty-four consecutive AF patients who underwent cardiac surgery to treat valvular or ischemic disease received concomitant Maze or mini-Maze ablation surgery with LAA AED placement. Patients were followed with a complete serial clinical status assessment, including computed tomographic (CT) scan, after 3 months and yearly thereafter up to 3 years after surgery. The authors reported a 100% effective LAA occlusion with no surgical learning curve, and no complications or neurologic events during follow-up. At 3-month follow-up, normal sinus rhythm was present in 70% of patients and AF was present in 20%. It also was found to be possible to perform an effective off-pump clip application in 15% of patients with paroxysmal AF who required pulmonary vein isolation and off-pump coronary artery bypass grafting.

In 2011, Benussi and colleagues[28] reported the first case of thoracoscopic appendage clip implantation as a solo procedure to treat an incessant drug-refractory atrial tachycardia in a 15-year-old boy who had previously undergone 2 failed percutaneous ablation attempts. A recently published study from Ohtsuka and colleagues[29] was specifically developed to evaluate the potential of stand-alone left atrial appendectomy to prevent TE in nonvalvular AF patients. Thirty patients with previous TE unsuitable for AOC received a thoracoscopic appendectomy and were followed for 38 months (mean 16 ± 9.7 months). The authors reported no mortality and no major postoperative complications. At 3-month follow-up, all patients discontinued warfarin and showed a complete excluded appendage on CT scans and, moreover, no one had experienced recurrence of TE.

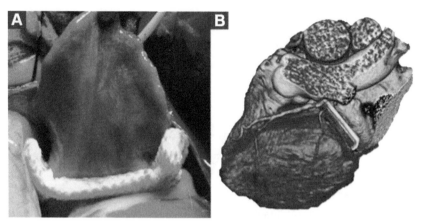

Fig. 8. (*A*) magnification of the excluded appendage. (*B*) Magnetic resonance imaging 3-dimensional rendering study showing that the device does not interfere with the surrounding structures of the heart. (Courtesy of Atri-Cure Inc, West Chester, OH.)

SUMMARY

Despite the promising results of these preliminary studies, further investigations involving carefully selected patients across a wider range of clinical settings will be necessary to answer important remaining questions. Can LAA occlusion devices be used to reduce stroke risk in both valvular and nonvalvular AF patients? If so, can it replace oral anticoagulation therapy? Are AEDs safe and effective in the long term?

To answer these and other important questions, 2 phase II clinical trials, the EXCLUDE trial (NCT00779857) and the Safety and Effectiveness of LAA Occlusion trial (NCT00567515), have been specifically designed.

Preliminary results from the former study, regarding safety and efficacy of the AED device, have already been published.[30] Seventy-one patients were enrolled at 7 different cardiothoracic US centers and received concomitant AtriClip device insertion. Authors reported a completely successful LAA exclusion rate, assessed at operation (by TEE) and at 3-month follow-up (by CT angiography or TEE), of 95.7% and 98.4%, respectively. After deployment, there was no evidence of clip migration. No adverse events related to the clip were reported, and none of the patients suffered from strokes or cardioembolic events at 6-month follow-up. Moreover, 70.3% of patients discontinued oral anticoagulants, at 12-month follow-up.

The long-term results from the NCT00567515 trial have recently been reported.[31] This single-center study enrolled 40 patients who underwent LAA occlusion concomitantly to an ablation procedure. Patients were followed up with electrocardiogram, chest radiograph, TEE, and CT studies 3 months after surgery and then yearly up to

3 years. The authors reported an early mortality of 10% because of non-device-related reasons with 32 patients completing all follow-up assessments. On CT, LAA clips were found to be completely occlusive and stable, showing no LAA reperfusion nor secondary dislocation in all patients. Only one episode of transient ischemic attack, recognized as of noncardiac origin, was reported in one patient 2 years after surgery. At 3-year follow-up time, 90.7% of patients discontinued oral anticoagulants.

These data suggest that exclusion of the LAA can be performed safely and without injury to the heart and surrounding structures during open cardiac surgery, with a high efficacy exclusion rate in short- and long-term follow-up. However, further investigations are necessary to define the role of this new device as a stand-alone therapy in the setting of stroke-prevention strategy.

Surgical therapies for stroke prevention continue to evolve. Patient demand for minimally invasive techniques will exponentially grow. Therefore, innovating and refining less invasive methods that focus on providing the superior results of the Cox-Maze procedure must be continued with endoscopic approaches that facilitate quicker patient recovery, faster healing, improved cosmetics, and overall lower patient morbidity.

VIDEOS

Videos related to this article can be found at http://dx.doi.org/10.1016/j.iccl.2013.12.004.

REFERENCES

1. Roger VL, Go AS, Lloyd-Jones DM, et al. Heart disease and stroke statistics–2012 update: a report

from the American Heart Association. Circulation 2012;125:e2–220.

2. Secondary prevention in non-rheumatic atrial fibrillation after transient ischaemic attack or minor stroke. EAFT (European Atrial Fibrillation Trial) Study Group. Lancet 1993;342:1255–62.

3. Waldo AL, Becker RC, Tapson VF, et al. Hospitalized patients with atrial fibrillation and a high risk of stroke are not being provided with adequate anticoagulation. J Am Coll Cardiol 2005;46:1729–36.

4. Blackshear JL, Odell JA. Appendage obliteration to reduce stroke in cardiac surgical patients with atrial fibrillation. Ann Thorac Surg 1996;61:755–9.

5. Al-Saady NM, Obel OA, Camm AJ. Left atrial appendage: structure, function, and role in thromboembolism. Heart 1999;82:547–54.

6. Agmon Y, Khandheria BK, Gentile F, et al. Echocardiographic assessment of the left atrial appendage. J Am Coll Cardiol 1999;34:1867–77.

7. Donal E, Yamada H, Leclercq C, et al. The left atrial appendage, a small, blind-ended structure: a review of its echocardiographic evaluation and its clinical role. Chest 2005;128:1853–62.

8. Heist EK, Refaat M, Danik SB, et al. Analysis of the left atrial appendage by magnetic resonance angiography in patients with atrial fibrillation. Heart Rhythm 2006;3:1313–8.

9. Hoit BD, Shao Y, Tsai LM, et al. Altered left atrial compliance after atrial appendectomy. Influence on left atrial and ventricular filling. Circ Res 1993;72:167–75.

10. Di Biase L, Burkhardt JD, Mohanty P, et al. Left atrial appendage: an underrecognized trigger site of atrial fibrillation. Circulation 2010;122:109–18.

11. Belcher JR, Somerville W. Systemic embolism and left auricular thrombosis in relation to mitral valvotomy. Br Med J 1955;2:1000–3.

12. Madden JL. Resection of the left auricular appendix; a prophylaxis for recurrent arterial emboli. J Am Med Assoc 1949;140:769–72.

13. Leonard FC, Cogan MA. Failure of ligation of the left auricular appendage in the prevention of recurrent embolism. N Engl J Med 1952;246:733–5.

14. Prasad SM, Maniar HS, Camillo CJ, et al. The Cox maze III procedure for atrial fibrillation: long-term efficacy in patients undergoing lone versus concomitant procedures. J Thorac Cardiovasc Surg 2003;126:1822–8.

15. Pet M, Robertson JO, Bailey M, et al. The impact of CHADS2 score on late stroke after the Cox maze procedure. J Thorac Cardiovasc Surg 2013;146:85–9.

16. Johnson WD, Ganjoo AK, Stone CD, et al. The left atrial appendage: our most lethal human attachment! Surgical implications. Eur J Cardiothorac Surg 2000;17:718–22.

17. Camm AJ, Kirchhof P, Lip GY, et al. Guidelines for the management of atrial fibrillation: the Task Force for the Management of Atrial Fibrillation of the European Society of Cardiology (ESC). Eur Heart J 2010;31:2369–429.

18. Bonow RO, Carabello BA, Chatterjee K, et al. ACC/AHA 2006 guidelines for the management of patients with valvular heart disease: a report of the American College of Cardiology/American Heart Association Task Force on Practice Guidelines (writing Committee to Revise the 1998 guidelines for the management of patients with valvular heart disease) developed in collaboration with the Society of Cardiovascular Anesthesiologists endorsed by the Society for Cardiovascular Angiography and Interventions and the Society of Thoracic Surgeons. J Am Coll Cardiol 2006;48:e1–148.

19. Healey JS, Crystal E, Lamy A, et al. Left Atrial Appendage Occlusion Study (LAAOS): results of a randomized controlled pilot study of left atrial appendage occlusion during coronary bypass surgery in patients at risk for stroke. Am Heart J 2005;150:288–93.

20. Garcia-Fernandez MA, Perez-David E, Quiles J, et al. Role of left atrial appendage obliteration in stroke reduction in patients with mitral valve prosthesis: a transesophageal echocardiographic study. J Am Coll Cardiol 2003;42:1253–8.

21. Kanderian AS, Gillinov AM, Pettersson GB, et al. Success of surgical left atrial appendage closure: assessment by transesophageal echocardiography. J Am Coll Cardiol 2008;52:924–9.

22. Wolf RK. Minimally invasive surgical treatment of atrial fibrillation. Semin Thorac Cardiovasc Surg 2007;19:311–8.

23. Blackshear JL, Johnson WD, Odell JA, et al. Thoracoscopic extracardiac obliteration of the left atrial appendage for stroke risk reduction in atrial fibrillation. J Am Coll Cardiol 2003;42:1249–52.

24. McCarthy PM, Lee R, Foley JL, et al. Occlusion of canine atrial appendage using an expandable silicone band. J Thorac Cardiovasc Surg 2010;140:885–9.

25. Fumoto H, Gillinov AM, Ootaki Y, et al. A novel device for left atrial appendage exclusion: the third-generation atrial exclusion device. J Thorac Cardiovasc Surg 2008;136:1019–27.

26. Salzberg SP, Gillinov AM, Anyanwu A, et al. Surgical left atrial appendage occlusion: evaluation of a novel device with magnetic resonance imaging. Eur J Cardiothorac Surg 2008;34:766–70.

27. Salzberg SP, Plass A, Emmert MY, et al. Left atrial appendage clip occlusion: early clinical results. J Thorac Cardiovasc Surg 2010;139:1269–74.

28. Benussi S, Mazzone P, Maccabelli G, et al. Thoracoscopic appendage exclusion with an atriclip device

as a solo treatment for focal atrial tachycardia. Circulation 2011;123:1575–8.

29. Ohtsuka T, Ninomiya M, Nonaka T, et al. Thoracoscopic stand-alone left atrial appendectomy for thromboembolism prevention in nonvalvular atrial fibrillation. J Am Coll Cardiol 2013;62:103–7.

30. Ailawadi G, Gerdisch MW, Harvey RL, et al. Exclusion of the left atrial appendage with a novel device:

early results of a multicenter trial. J Thorac Cardiovasc Surg 2011;142:1002–9, 1009.e1.

31. Emmert MY, Puippe G, Baumuller S, et al. Safe, effective and durable epicardial left atrial appendage clip occlusion in patients with atrial fibrillation undergoing cardiac surgery: first long-term results from a prospective device trial. Eur J Cardiothorac Surg 2013;45(1):126–31.

Device- and LAA-Specific Characteristics for Successful LAA Closure: Tips and Tricks

Wen-Loong Yeow, MD[a], Saibal Kar, MD[a,b],*

KEYWORDS

- Nonvalvular atrial fibrillation • Ischemic embolic strokes
- Transcatheter left atrial appendage occlusion

KEY POINTS

- Endovascular closure and epicardial ligation of the left atrial appendage (LAA) are clinically feasible alternatives to oral anticoagulation for nonvalvular atrial fibrillation.
- Transcatheter LAA closure is intuitive, because no appendages are the same.
- There are tips and tricks for transcatheter LAA closure that will reduce the learning curve and improve procedural results.

INTRODUCTION

Since the introduction of left atrial appendage (LAA) closure for stroke prevention in patients with nonvalvular atrial fibrillation (AF), several devices and approaches have been developed to achieve optimal closure. Although the procedural steps for each device are intuitive, methodical, and systematic, there are tips and tricks at each step necessary for the varied LAA anatomy and device characteristics.

The functional anatomy of the LAA and the recommended site of closure are discussed first. The salient steps of the procedure and associated tips and tricks are then discussed according to each device and applicability to a range of LAA. These steps include overcoming challenges in transseptal and LAA access, image correlation and appropriate working views, device selection, and deployment. The 4 devices that are covered are the WATCHMAN, AMPLATZER Cardiac Plug, Coherex WaveCrest generation 1.3, and the LARIAT suture delivery device.

THE FUNCTIONAL ANATOMY OF THE LAA

The LAA can be divided into the proximal "neck" and the functional LAA (**Fig. 1**A). The smooth walled neck is derived from the pulmonary veins while the trabeculated functional LAA is derived from the primordial left atrium and is the principal site for thrombus formation. The ostium of the functional LAA is usually located at the level of the circumflex artery. This ostium is ideally suited for device deployment, because closure at this level will isolate the thrombus source of the LAA. In addition, the tubular shape from the ostium onwards provides circumferential support and ensures device stability. In comparison, support from the 3-dimensional spiral configuration of the neck is inadequate and device deployment at this level is not recommended (**Fig. 2**A). Incidentally, the frequently observed pits along the neck

Conflict of Interest: S. Kar has received research grants from Boston Scientific, St. Jude Medical, and Coherex. W.L. Yeow has no relationships relevant to the contents of this article to disclose.
[a] Heart Institute, Cedars-Sinai Medical Center, 8631 West Third Street, Los Angeles, CA 90048, USA; [b] David Geffen School of Medicine at UCLA, Los Angeles, CA 90095, USA
* Corresponding author. Heart Institute, Cedars-Sinai Medical Center, 8631 West Third Street, Room 415E, Los Angeles, CA 90048.
E-mail address: karsk@cshs.org

Intervent Cardiol Clin 3 (2014) 239–254
http://dx.doi.org/10.1016/j.iccl.2013.12.002
2211-7458/14/$ – see front matter © 2014 Elsevier Inc. All rights reserved.

interventional.theclinics.com

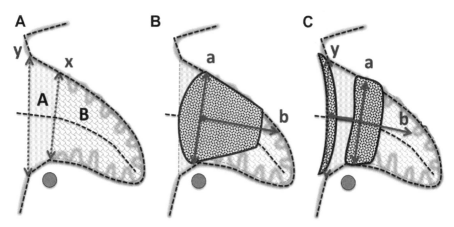

Fig. 1. (*A*) Stylized diagram depicting the proximal "neck" (zone A) and its opening (y), and the functional trabeculated LAA (zone B) and its ostium (x). (*B*) The WATCHMAN device size (a) is determined by the maximal ostial width (x) and is ideally deployed at the ostium. The depth (b) measured from the ostium ensures the distal tines of the WATCHMAN device can be accommodated. (*C*) The AMPLATZER cardiac plug device size (a) is determined by the maximum width of the opening (y), while the depth (b) ensures there is adequate depth for the device to provide sufficient retraction on the disc. The body of the AMPLATZER cardiac plug is ideally deployed at the ostium (x).

are unlikely sources of thrombus and do not require occlusion (see **Fig. 2**B).

THE WATCHMAN DEVICE

The WATCHMAN device (Atritech, a subsidiary of Boston Scientific, Plymouth, MN, USA), a self-expanding device (nitinol frame) with a polyethylene terephthalate cover and fixation barbs on its side, is probably the most familiar system in use. The major advantage with this system is that it has the largest published data to date and, because there is only one lobe, is relatively intuitive to deploy.[1] Its major limitations are the pointed distal tines and the device is not redeployable once it has been fully recaptured. Future

generations are being developed to address these issues.

The current generation of WATCHMAN sizes and lengths are summarized in **Table 1**. The required device size is determined by the maximal width at the level of the circumflex artery and perpendicular to the trajectory of the access sheath (AS) (see **Fig. 1**B). A thorough transesophageal echocardiographic (TEE) assessment is required to determine the maximum dimensions; the largest widths are often measured in the 0° and 135° TEE views. Simultaneous biplane function of the TEE probe is effective at producing orthogonal views for LAA assessment; the measured widths should be at the corresponding height in the orthogonal plane (**Fig. 3**).

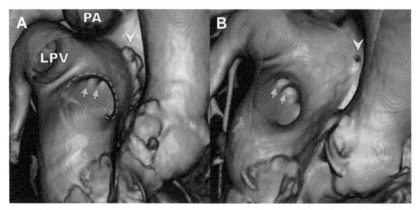

Fig. 2. (*A*) The neck of the appendage has a 3-dimensional spiral configuration (*dotted line*). (*B*) Pits are commonly observed in the neck of the appendage (*arrows*). The tip of the appendage (*arrowhead*) is posterior to the aorta. LPV, left pulmonary vein; PA, pulmonary artery.

Table 1
The WATCHMAN device sizing chart and dimensions (The compression diameters guide post deployment stability assessment)

Maximum Width (mm)	Device Size (mm)	Device Length (mm)	Acceptable Compression Diameters (mm)
17–19	21	20.2	16.8–19.3
20–22	24	22.9	19.2–22.1
23–25	27	26.5	21.6–24.8
26–28	30	29.4	24.0–27.6
29–31	33	31.6	26.4–30.4

The chosen device should be 3 to 4 mm larger than the maximum width. In cases where the left atrial (LA) pressure is low (<10 mm Hg), additional fluids should be administered to the patients, and the widths should be repeated. This essential step avoids undersizing and embolization of a device. Erring on the larger device prevents undersizing for measurement in between sizes. An en faced TEE probe during final measurements prevents undersizing (**Fig. 4**).

Transseptal Puncture and LAA Access

LA access via a transseptal puncture (TSP) is one of the most critical steps in the procedure. A correctly performed and located TSP helps orientates the AS along the long axis of the LAA and thereby promotes proper device deployment and orientation. Accordingly, the anatomic location of the ostium and orientation of the LAA, as well as the type of catheters used to access the LAA, dictates the site of puncture. As most LAAs are located in the left superior-anterior section of the LA and pointed in a lateral anterior-superior direction, the TSP for LAA closure should be the middle to inferior/posterior aspect of the fossa (**Fig. 5A**).[2]

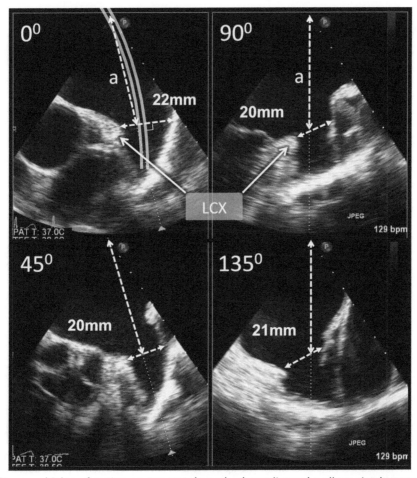

Fig. 3. Simultaneous biplane function on transesophageal echocardiography allows simultaneous orthogonal assessment of the LAA. The maximal widths are measured perpendicular to the trajectory of the AS (*double line*) at the level of the left circumflex artery and at the corresponding height (a) in the orthogonal plane.

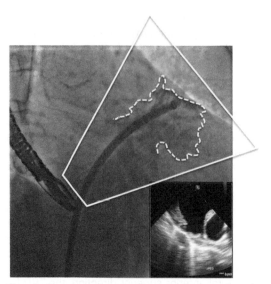

Fig. 4. Fluoroscopic-assisted transesophageal echo probe direction for an en face assessment (*inset*) of the LAA (*dotted line*) ostium.

An inferior-posterior TSP site is ideal for most WATCHMAN procedures. This site maintains alignment with the long axis of the LAA while the AS is placed at the required depth to accommodate the device (see **Fig. 5**B). An anterior or superior puncture aligns the AS across the long axis of the LAA (see **Fig. 5**C, D). To realign the AS, retracting and then advancement with counterclockwise rotation may direct it along the long axis of the LAA.

To achieve an accurate TSP, reliance on fluoroscopy alone is insufficient. The combination of TEE and fluoroscopy with or without an integrated system such as Philips' Echonavigator live image guidance tool are advantageous; TEE-guided TSP facilitates accurate localization, avoiding punctures through the posterior wall or roof of the LA, and assists in the early detection of a pericardial effusion. In addition, the simultaneous biplane function aligned to the tip of the dilator during septal tenting facilitates accurate short- and long-axis localization before puncturing (**Fig. 6**).

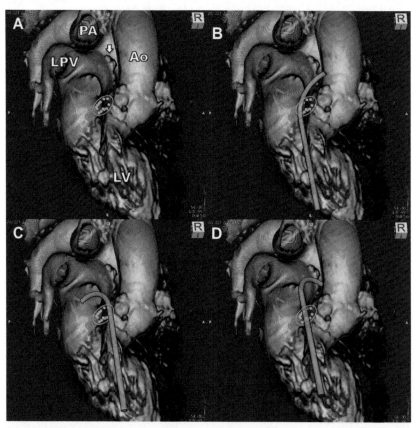

Fig. 5. (*A*) Endocardial view of the left atrium from a 3-dimensional CT image. The location of the fossa ovalis (*green dots*) was marked from the axial slices. The tip of the LAA (*arrow*) is posterior to the aorta. (*B*) An inferior and posterior TSP facilitates a single curve AS into the LAA. (*C*) An anterior puncture directs a single curve AS posteriorly across the ostial face. (*D*) A superior puncture directs the single curve AS inferiorly across the ostial face. Ao, aorta; LPV, left pulmonary vein; LV, left ventricle; PA, pulmonary artery.

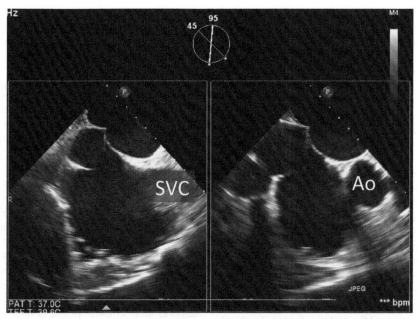

Fig. 6. Simultaneous biplane transesophageal assessment of the transseptal sheath tenting the septum in the bicaval (90°–100°) and aortic valve short-axis (35°–50°) view. Ao, aorta; SVC, superior vena cava.

Reshaping the Brockenbrough transseptal needle by increasing the acuity of the distal curve improves septal tenting and reduces the risk of the needle tip slipping during punctures. However a longer curve needle may provide extra reach with bulging septum toward the left atrium. Conversely, bulging septum toward the right atrium displaces a nominal curved needle less than an acutely angle curve.

Resistance to needle puncture is often due to increased septal thickness or scarring from previous punctures. Further resistance to puncture corresponds to the thicker edge of the fossa ovalis during inferior posterior punctures. Excessive traction on the septum is sine qua non of an unsuccessful puncture (**Fig. 7**). Puncturing with the needle stylet or the stiff end of a 0.014-inch coronary angioplasty wire, or tapping the shaft of the needle with an electrosurgical device set at cauterization, can overcome the resistance.

Following successful TSP, intravenous heparin is given, aiming for an activated clotting time

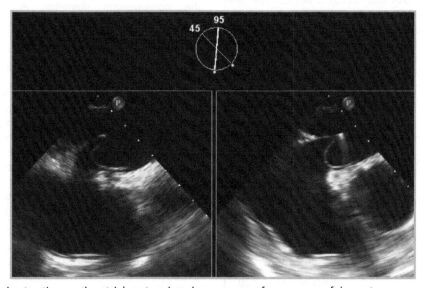

Fig. 7. Excessive traction on the atrial septum is a sine qua non of an unsuccessful puncture.

greater than 250 seconds. An SL1 transseptal sheath (St. Jude Medical, Minneapolis, MN, USA) is preferable over a standard Mullins sheath because it is easier to advance into the pulmonary vein. The straight rail over a short tipped (1 cm) superstiff exchange length wire provides strong support for large-caliber sheaths or catheter exchanges across the atrial septum.

Selecting a single- or double-curve AS partially depends on the operator's preference. The distal curve of the double-curve AS is orthogonal to the proximal curve and provides additional anterior-superior directionality. It is useful as an all-purpose catheter especially for superiorly orientated LAA. A single-curve catheter can be equally useful providing the TSP location is inferior-posterior.

Access into the LAA with a pigtail catheter reduces the risk of perforation. Through the AS a 5-Fr pigtail catheter is rotated superiorly (counterclockwise rotation) and advanced into the LAA and then used as a rail for the AS (the AS should not be advanced past the pigtail catheter). To select the anterior or posterior lobe, the pigtail is rotated counterclockwise or clockwise, respectively, before advancement. For difficult LAA access an angulated pigtail catheter provides additional directionality.

The Working View

Interpreting and marrying the LAA views on TEE and fluoroscopy are vital for device deployment. The corresponding TEE and fluoroscopic views are summarized in **Table 2**. Although initial access into the LAA is often performed with the anterior-posterior (AP) fluoroscopic view, a corresponding TEE-fluoroscopic view is required to evaluate the LAA and deploy a device. The best working view depends on the information required. Generally the best TEE working views are the 45° and 135° views; the profile of the left lateral ridge is demonstrated in the 45° view while the 135° view separates the anterior and posterior lobes of most LAA (**Fig. 8**). Consequently the right anterior-oblique (RAO) cranial and RAO caudal

are the best fluoroscopic working views. To marry the views, the TEE view is rotated 180°. The working view for the WATCHMAN device is the RAO 30°, caudal 20°, and 135° TEE views.

Device Deployment, Recapture, and Release

Once the device size has been selected, the corresponding position along the proximal radiopaque markers of the AS is aligned to the ostium, ensuring adequate depth is available (**Fig. 9**A). With the device loaded, the AS straightens and a greater anterior-superior position maybe attained (see **Fig. 9**B). To reduce the risk of device perforation, the respirator is slowed or held as the WATCHMAN is deployed. As the device is unsheathed, the position of the distal tines is maintained by holding the deployment knob (see **Fig. 9**C). Following deployment, the distal tines recoil away from the LAA and the device settles perpendicular to the alignment of the AS (see **Fig. 9**D). For larger devices a second step in deployment is essential to avoid dislodgment; as the proximal frame is unsheathed, the sudden and forceful expansion, if unanticipated, can eject the delivery system and device. To prevent this, a counterforce is applied to the deployment knob, as the proximal frame is unsheathed.

Assessments of device stability (through a tug test and final compression size) and closure success (through shoulder height and color Doppler assessments) are crucial before device release. Stability on a tug test is confirmed when the appendage moves with the device. The tug should be firm, but not abrupt nor too soft. The final compression size is measured with the threaded insert in view, which prevents overestimation of the compression diameter. An acceptable compression is a diameter 80% to 92% of the original device size (see **Table 1**). As the polyethylene terephthalate covers half the device along its side, the acceptable shoulder height is equivalent to half the length of the device.

Recapturing the device to reorientate or correct a distal deployment requires partial recapture; the deployment knob is held firmly in the palm of the right hand while the thumb pushes the hub of the Y-connector, advancing the AS over the covered cap. For a device that protrudes excessively into the LA or a different size is required, a full recapture of the barbs and distal tines is performed; however, redeployment of the device is precluded.

Difficult LAA Anatomies

The shape of the LAA is less of a concern for most endocardial closure devices; for suitable ostial widths between 17 and 31 mm, the lack of depth

Table 2
Corresponding transesophageal echo and fluoroscopic views

Transesophageal Echo View	Fluoroscopic View
0°	AP cranial
45°	RAO 30°, cranial 20°
90°	RAO 30°
135°	RAO 30°, caudal 20°

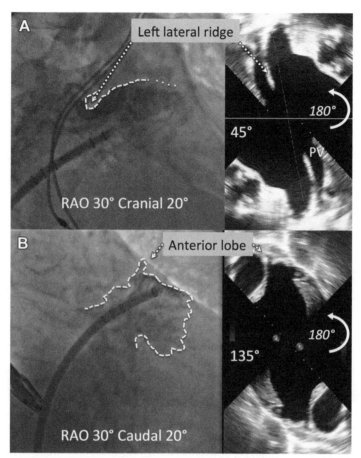

Fig. 8. Correlating fluoroscopic and transesophageal images in the 2 most useful working views. (*A*) The RAO cranial and 45° TEE views profile the left lateral ridge (*dotted line*). (*B*) The RAO caudal and 135° TEE views separate the anterior and posterior lobes (the *dotted line* outlines the LAA). To marry the views, the TEE image is rotated 180°. PV, pulmonary vein.

is concerning for the WATCHMAN device (**Fig. 10**). Aside from the risk of perforation from the distal tines, the deployed device may protrude excessively into the LA (**Fig. 11**). Aligning the AS and deploying the device into the anterior lobe reduces the inferior shoulder and permits a deeper deployment. Selective engagement of the anterior lobe is achieved through counterclockwise rotation of the AS and delivery system during advancement.

Summary

The principal procedural steps with the WATCHMAN device can be applied to most endocardial devices. Attention to device sizing, deployment, and pre-release criteria is essential to maximize procedural efficacy.

THE AMPLATZER CARDIAC PLUG

The disc of the AMPLATZER cardiac plug (AGA; St. Jude Medical) is designed to cap off the neck, while

the lobe anchors the device at the ostium of the functional LAA, also known as the "landing zone" (see **Fig. 1**C). The connecting flexible waist permits independent alignment of the disc and lobe and facilitates apposition to the orifice by retracting the disc. The device size is determined by the maximum width of the neck and a depth greater than 10 mm is required to accommodate the device (**Table 3**). Like the WATCHMAN device, the cardiac plug is not redeployable once it is fully recaptured.

The pivotal trial comparing the efficacy of the device with anticoagulation therapy is currently underway.[3] A second-generation device, the AMPLATZER Amulet, is available for clinical assessment; however, the discussion henceforth is limited to the Cardiac Plug.

TSP And LAA Access

An inferiorly located TSP is ideal for the cardiac plug. The AMPLATZER TorqVue 45° by 45° delivery sheath (DS) is designed to deploy the relatively

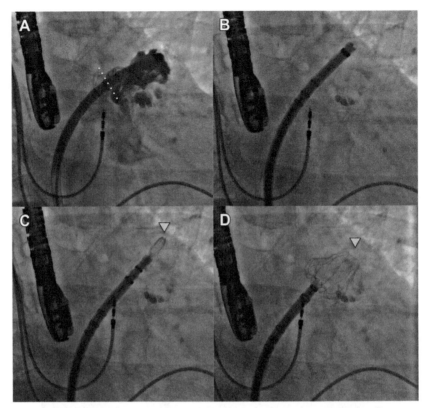

Fig. 9. (*A*) The selected device size and its corresponding length along the proximal radiopaque marker band when aligned to the ostium (*dotted line*) ensure adequate depth is available. (*B*) With the device loaded, the AS straightens, attaining a greater anterior-superior direction. (*C*) As the device is unsheathed, it is essential that the position of the distal tines (*triangle*) be maintained. (*D*) The distal tines (*triangle*) of the deployed device contract toward the covered cap and ostium.

shorter device at a shallower depth; the inferior TSP facilitates alignment of the DS along the long axis of the landing zone.

A marker pigtail catheter is required to access the LAA and assess its size. Following an angiogram of the LAA, the ostial width, landing zone, and depth are measured in the RAO 30°, cranial 20°, and caudal 20° views (**Fig. 12**A). As the recommended device size is based on the maximal ostial measurement, a quality angiogram of the LAA is crucial. Further assessments of the maximal widths and depths on the 0°, 45°, 90°, and 135° TEE views are performed to confirm device selection (see **Fig. 12**B). With the pigtail as the rail, the DS is advanced to the required depth (at least 10 mm from the ostium) and rotated (usually counterclockwise) in alignment with the landing zone. As the DS lacks radiopaque marker bands to guide depth placement, a referenced image of a measured angiogram of the LAA is a practical solution.

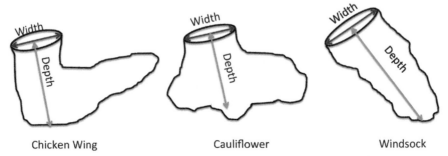

Chicken Wing   Cauliflower   Windsock

Fig. 10. LAA shape is less concerning than width and depth for endocardial closure devices.

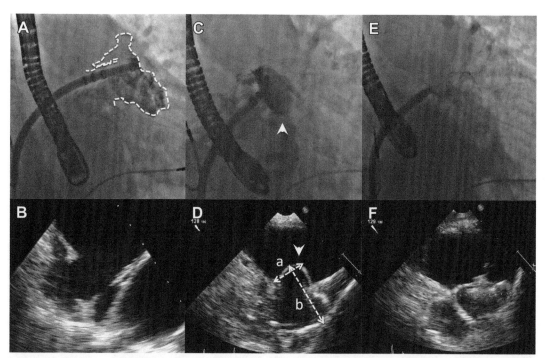

Fig. 11. (*A, B*) A LAA (*dotted line*) with a depth less than its width (short and wide body) can be difficult to close. (*C, D*) Inadvertent deployment into the posterior lobe leads to an inferior shoulder (*arrowhead*) with an unacceptable height (a) and insufficient compression (b). (*E, F*) Redeployment into the anterior lobe reduces the inferior shoulder.

The Working View

The RAO 30°, cranial 20°, and 45° TEE projections are ideal working views because the left pulmonary ridge can be visualized in profile (see **Fig. 8**A). Proximal deployment of the disc encroaching the pulmonary vein can be identified in these views.

Device Deployment, Recapture, and Release

Deploying the cardiac plug is a 3-step process; the first and second steps involve the deployment of the distal and proximal aspect of the lobe, respectively, and the third for the disc. The distal lobe is unsheathed below the level of the circumflex artery and about 10 mm distal from the ostium into the "ball configuration" (see **Fig. 12**C). The stabilizing wires are partially retracted in this configuration. Final adjustment in depth and directionality (maintaining the DS alignment with the landing zone) can be performed before the rest of the lobe is deployed. Advancing the delivery cable deploys the rest of lobe. At least two-thirds of the lobe should be distal to the circumflex artery (see **Fig. 12**D, E). A lobe deployed too proximal is at risk of embolization and does not provide adequate retraction on the disc, leading to a risk of incomplete ostial

Table 3
AMPLATZER cardiac plug device sizing chart and dimensions

Maximum Width (mm)	Device Size (mm)	Disc Diameter (mm)	Lobe Length (mm)	Waist Length (mm)
12.6–14.5	16	20	6.5	4
14.6–16.5	18	22		
16.6–18.5	20	24		
18.6–20.5	22	26		
20.6–22.5	24	30		
22.6–24.5	26	32		
24.6–26.5	28	34		
26.6–28.5	30	36		

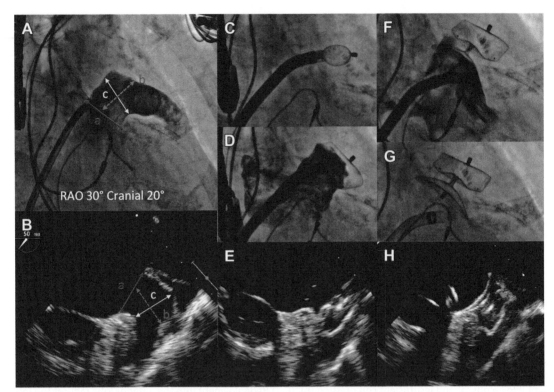

Fig. 12. (*A*) The ostial width (a), depth (b), and device size (c) measured on the angiogram of the LAA are calibrated to the marker pigtail. The tip of the DS should be positioned at least 10 mm distal to the ostium. (*B*) Confirming the ostial width (a), depth (b), and device size (c) on transesophageal echocardiography in a similar projection. (*C*) Deployment of the distal lobe into the "ball configuration." (*D*, *E*) Confirming the deployed lobe is at least two-thirds distal to the circumflex artery. (*F–H*) Closure is checked with contrast angiography and disc retraction, and the tire-shaped lobe is confirmed before the device can be released.

occlusion. Similarly a lobe deployed at depths more than 15 mm can be overly compressed, disengaging the stabilizing wires and pulling the disc into and mal-coapting with the proximal appendage. In addition, distal deployment may lead to LAA perforation and thrombus formation.

The third step is to deploy the disc; slight tension is applied to the delivery cable while the disc is unsheathed. Advancing the delivery cable (or DS) onto the deployed disc promotes symmetric concavity. Before the device is released, the shape, position, alignment, residual gaps, and separation of disc and lobe are assessed (**Fig. 12**F–H). The shape of the disc and lobe should be concave and tirelike, respectively (**Fig. 13**). The position and alignment of lobe in the landing zone and assessment of closure are performed with color Doppler (in 0°, 45°, 90°, and 135° views) and contrast fluoroscopy (RAO cranial and caudal views). In addition, mitral valve and pulmonary vein flows are also assessed for impingement. A tug test can be performed to confirm stability.

Recapturing and redeployment of the disc, to correct a tilted disc or incomplete closure, can be performed independently of the lobe. To recapture the disc, the delivery cable is held while the sheath is advanced. Rotating the DS counterclockwise will orientate the disc along the axis of the opening. If closure remains unsatisfactory, or the lobe is deployed in a tilted position or at an inappropriate depth, recapturing the lobe into the ball configuration is required. The delivery cable is held while the sheath is advanced until the platinum markers on the lobe are just distal to the radiopaque marker of the DS (**Fig. 14**). Counterclockwise rotation of the DS reorientates the lobe anterior superiorly and in parallel with the landing zone. Officially no more than 2 recaptures are recommended before replacement of the DS and device is required.

Difficult LAA Anatomies

Compared with the WATCHMAN device, the Cardiac Plug is suited to short broad appendages. However, to accommodate the device, a minimal depth of 10 mm is required. Tortuous LAA may present a challenge, because aligning the DS in

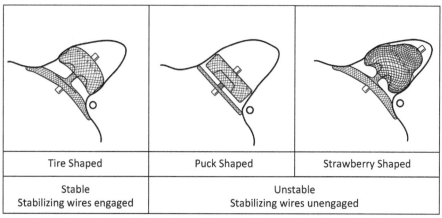

Tire Shaped	Puck Shaped	Strawberry Shaped
Stable	Unstable	
Stabilizing wires engaged	Stabilizing wires unengaged	

Fig. 13. The shape of the disc and lobe is assessed for stability before the device is released. (*Reprinted from* St. Jude Medical, St. Paul, MN, © 2013 All rights reserved; with permission.)

parallel with the landing may be difficult. However, in most cases rotating the DS counterclockwise into the LAA improves alignment and orientating the device en face with the landing zone.

Summary

The location of the TSP, thorough assessment of the LAA dimension, alignment of the DS with

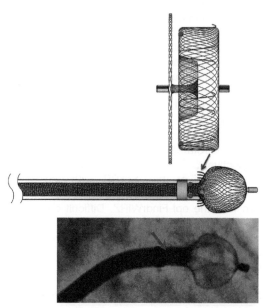

Fig. 14. Partial deployment of the lobe, the "ball configuration," is confirmed on fluoroscopy once the platinum thread markers (*red dots*) are aligned just distal (*red arrow*) to the radiopaque marker band on the DS. Importantly, this configuration prevents damage to the sheath during partial recapture as the stabilizing wires (*purple arrow*) remains distal to the sheath. (*Reprinted from* St. Jude Medical, St. Paul, MN, © 2013 All rights reserved; with permission.)

the landing zone, and assessing the closure and shape of the device are essential to achieve optimal procedural results.

THE COHEREX WAVECREST

The Coherex WaveCrest generation 1.3 device (Coherex Medical, Salt Lake City, UT, USA) is a completely retrievable, repositionable, and redeployable system consisting of an occluding cap and anchoring wires. The early safety results have been promising, suggesting the device is safe and effective.[4] The occlusive cap is covered with expanded polytetrafluoroethylene (ePTFE), a material with low thrombogenicity, and is surrounded by polyurethane foam. When the constraint device is unsheathed, the foamed leading edge reduces the risk of perforation. The anchoring nitinol wires roll out to anchor the unsheathed cap and rolls in to allow for repositioning and recapturing.

Determining the maximal LAA ostium (at the level of the circumflex artery) on TEE need not be precise because there are only 3 sizes. The standard working views are the RAO 30°, cranial 20°, and 45° TEE views.

Once again, a targeted TSP to the inferior and posterior aspect of the fossa ovalis and using the left pulmonary vein for sheath exchanges are essential procedural steps (see above). Deep engagement of the LAA is not required. A standard pigtail is required for LAA access and as a rail for the DS. The DS is inserted just distal to the landing zone and rotated (usually counterclockwise) in alignment with the neck. Deployment is a 2-step procedure: unsheathing the foamed leading edge cover and then rolling out the distal anchors. At the end of each step, position and orientation of the device are confirmed on contrast angiography and TEE images. As the low thrombogenic ePTFE cover is occlusive, contrast can be injected through the hub to determine the final position and stability during tug test.

To reposition the device, retracting the anchor actuator rolls the distal anchors away from the appendage wall and into the cover, allowing the cover to be manipulated into position. Further retraction of the cover into the sheath allows the device to be fully repositionable and redeployable. Following confirmation of ostial closure and device stability, the device can be release. During detachment, the releasing mechanism prevents transfer of the torque and the position of the device is not disrupted.

The combination of the low thrombogenic ePTFE cover with a foam leading edge and retractable anchors should translate to a reduction in procedural complications and device-related thrombus formation. It is anticipated a larger trial with longer follow-ups will continue to support these design features.

THE LARIAT SUTURE DELIVERY DEVICE

The LARIAT suture delivery device (SentreHEART, Inc, Redwood City, CA, USA) resolves the risks of device embolization and thrombogenicity by ligating the LAA through an epicardial approach. The procedural steps require a thorough understanding of the device and its limitations. The key steps include preprocedural planning with computed tomographic (CT) scan, pericardial access, endo-FindrWIRZ positioning, and alignment of the snare.

Role of CT Scan

A cardiac CT scan is required to assess the LAA anatomy and determine its suitability for the LARIAT device. Its 40-mm pretied suture loop limits the size of the LAA that can be accommodated. The maximal width of the LAA, also known as the barrel width, is measured on an equivalent left anterior-oblique (LAO) 30° view. An LAA with lobes that fold back on it (ie, chicken wing–shaped LAA) or have a distal tip behind the pulmonary artery is excluded. In addition, the direction, steepness, and depth of the pericardial puncture can be preplanned and the anterior-superior LAA lobe can be identified and referenced during the procedure (**Fig. 15**).

Pericardial Access

Aside from gaining access to the pericardium, the directionality of the skin to pericardial punctures facilitates alignment of the epicardial components

with the LAA. Failure to connect the FindrWIRZ or to snare the LAA can result from misalignment. A Tuohy shaped epidural needle is ideally suited for the pericardial access. Pericardial access is performed via the subxiphoid approach. The puncture is 1 to 2 cm below and left of the lower edge of the sternum. The direction in the AP fluoroscopic view is toward the left shoulder and the puncture is performed in the lateral fluoroscopic view. The steepness of the puncture is kept shallow; steep punctures greater than 15° angulate the SofTIP, distorting the directionality, and can rotate the LARIAT device as it is advance through it.

Confirming pericardial access can be achieved with contrast boluses or with a J-tipped wire; looping and crossing the midline with the wire confirms pericardial access. Dilating the skin ensures the SofTIP does not crumple like a concertina as it is advanced. The SofTIP is inserted with the marked surface facing upwards (12 o'clock position) and then rotated toward the operator (9 o'clock position) as the tip approaches the LAA. The guidewire is left in place, safeguarding inadvertent displacement of the SofTIP.

Endo-FindrWIRZ Positioning

The TSP is performed at the mid fossa and an angled pigtail catheter promotes access of the SL1 sheath into the LAA. A quality angiogram of the LAA in the 2 working views, the RAO 30°, caudal 20°, and LAO 30° views, ensures all the major lobes are recognized, enabling correct identification of the anterior-superior lobe. Curving the tip of the endo-FindrWIR expedites placement in the preferred lobe. An angiogram of the LAA is repeated to confirm placement and depth. To reposition the endo-FindrWIRZ anteriorly or posteriorly, it is rotated counterclockwise or clockwise, respectively.

Alignment of the SofTIP with the endo-FindrWIRZ in the LAO 30° view assures connection with the epi-FindrWIRZ. Difficult connection due to anterior or posterior misalignment can be corrected by rotating the SofTIP counterclockwise or clockwise, respectively (opposite to endocardial rotation) (**Fig. 16**).

Snare Alignment, Deployment, and Removal

The LARIAT device is inserted with the flat face of the handle aligned to the SofTIP's marked surface (**Fig. 17**), ensuring the curves of the 2 components are aligned and the snare exits the SofTIP with the radiopaque marker on the left side in the LAO 30° projection (**Fig. 18**A, B). A right-sided marker position represents a rotated "upside down" LARIAT, a position not conducive to

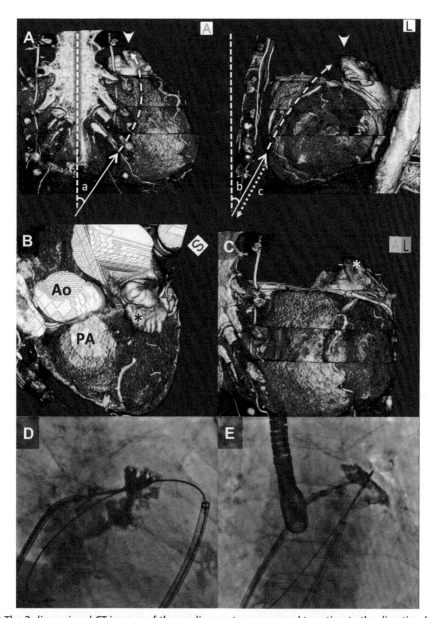

Fig. 15. (*A*) The 3-dimensional CT images of the cardiac anatomy are used to estimate the direction (a), steepness (b), and depth (c) of the TSP aligned to the LAA (*arrowhead*). The location of the anterior-superior lobe (*asterisk*) in the superior (*B*) and anterior-lateral (*C*) 3-dimensional CT images are referenced during angiograms of the LAA to ensure it is selected in the RAO 30°, caudal 20° (*D*), and LAO 30° (*E*) projections. Ao, aorta; PA, pulmonary artery.

snaring (see **Fig. 18C**), often the result of a steep pericardial puncture. Reducing the steepness by flattening the stomach may improve the malrotation. If this is unsuccessful and before another pericardial access is attempted, inserting the LARIAT with the flat face of the handle away from the SofTIP's marked surface may counterrotate the marker to the correct side.

The snare is then opened and brought up and over the LAA. With multilobed appendages, the anterior and then the posterior lobe is enveloped. Rotating the handle clockwise while advancing captures the anterior lobe and then counterclockwise while advancing captures the posterior lobe. The snare is then brought up to the level of the circumflex artery as marked by the EndoCATH balloon. To ensure the snare has not rotated, the radiopaque marker is maintained to the left in the RAO 30°, caudal 20° view (see **Fig. 18D, E**). If the snare is upside down with the marker to the right,

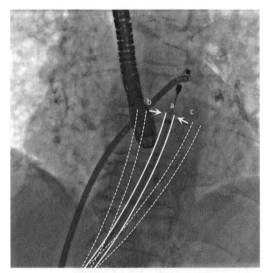

Fig. 16. Alignment of the SofTIP (a) with the anterior-superior lobe of the LAA in the LAO 30° projection assures connection of the FindrWIRZ. To correct an anterior (b) or posterior (c) misalignment the SofTIP is rotated counterclockwise or clockwise, respectively.

rotating the LARIAT to correct the orientation is performed before the snare can be closed.

Aspiration through the lumen of the EndoCATH once the snare is closed may reduce the volume and size of the LAA and assist removal of the snare. Once the snare is closed, the endo-FindrWIRZ and EndoCATH are retracted into the transseptal sheath and the suture is tightened with 10 lbs of force as marked on the TenSURE device. Repeating the suture tightening can close residual leaks detected on contrast angiography or color Doppler TEE. The proximal

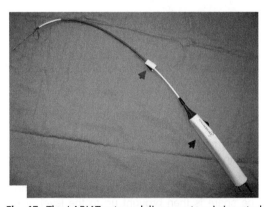

Fig. 17. The LARIAT suture delivery system is inserted with the flat part of the handle (*blue arrow*) aligned to the marked surface of the SofTIP (*red arrow*), thus ensuring the curves of both components are matched. (*Courtesy of* SentreHeart, Redwood City, CA; with permission.)

suture end is designed to come off the TenSURE device at 13 lbs of force and can be retied if further tightening is required.

The snare is then opened fully at the level of ligation before it is retracted. During retraction, a hang-up of the snare on fluoroscopy or resistance suggests a lobe is ensnared and further retraction may avulse the LAA. To release the ensnared lobe, the snare is brought back to the level of the ligation and opened and closed a few times.

The epi-FindrWIRZ is relocated into its trough before the 2 components can be retracted into the SofTIP; the combined widths can trap both components within SofTIP (**Fig. 19**). First the epi-FindrWIRZ is retracted to the tip of the SofTIP followed by the open snare and finally advancing the epi-FindrWIRZ into the snare ensures its relocation back into the trough. Once the 2 components are removed, the suture is cut (with the SureCUT device) and the SofTIP is replaced with a pigtail drainage catheter.

Summary

There are many aspects of the LARIAT procedure that are different than the endovascular closure technique. As no endovascular device is implanted, the risk of embolization and device thrombus is nonexistent. Understanding the key steps (see above) is essential for procedure success.

MANAGING COMPLICATIONS
Femoral Vein Access Hemostasis

As with most procedures requiring full anticoagulation, achieving access hemostasis is essential for patient comfort and preventing procedural complications. A subcutaneous figure-of-8 stitch can achieve immediate hemostasis despite the size of sheath used.[5] A thick silk suture (for example, a 0-0 silk suture) is passed subcutaneously under and then over the large sheath, then subcutaneously again, forming a "Z." The ends are tied into a fisherman's knot and tightened as the sheath is removed. Following 4 hours of bed rest, the suture is removed; as re-bleeds may occur (sitting and standing increase venous pressure), a short period of observation is required. Alternatively, a single Perclose Proglide Suture-Mediated Closure System (Abbott Vascular, Abbott Park, IL, USA) could be used off-label to achieve venous access hemostasis.

LAA Perforation

Extravasation of contrast into the pericardium or hemodynamic instability during catheter or device

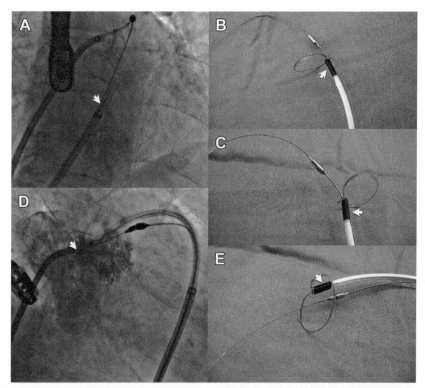

Fig. 18. (*A*) The position of the radiopaque marker (*arrow*) on the snare is checked in the LAO 30° projection as it exits the SofTIP. (*B*) A left-sided marker position (*arrow*) indicates a correctly orientated snare. (*C*) A right-sided marker position (*arrow*) indicates an inverted snare that is not conducive for snaring the LAA. (*D*) The position of the marker (*arrow*) on the snare is checked in the RAO 30°, caudal 20° projection before it is closed. (*E*) A left-sided marker position (*arrow*) indicates a correctly orientated snare. (*Courtesy of* SentreHeart, Redwood City, CA; with permission.)

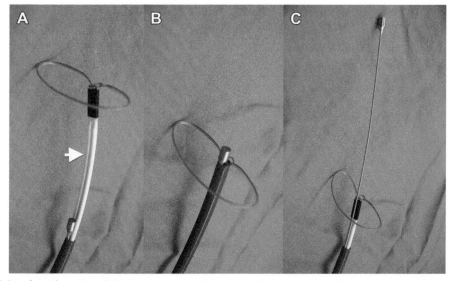

Fig. 19. (*A*) Before the epicardial components can be removed, the operator first retracts the epi-FindrWIRZ to the SofTIP, relocating it within its trough (*arrow*). (*B*) The snare is then brought down to the tip. (*C*) Finally, the epi-FindrWIRZ is advanced, then the snare, and with the snare closed both components are removed together. (*Courtesy of* SentreHeart, Redwood City, CA; with permission.)

manipulations within the LAA is phenotypical of a perforation. Deploying the endovascular device or completing the epicardial ligation should seal the perforation. Pericardiocentesis is then performed with reinfusion of the aspirated blood. In anticipation of pericardiocentesis, a 4-Fr femoral vein sheath can be inserted at time of femoral vein access.

Air Embolism

Prevention of air embolism is imperative. Preparations of the ASs and delivery system with ample flushes of heparinized saline are essential. Continuous flushing of the delivery system with the sidearm connected to the manifold during insertion into the AS ensures an air-free connection. Aspiration of the AS and delivery system is avoided because air may be drawn into the system through the proximal valve.

Incomplete Closure

Incomplete closures with large gaps detected on follow-up TEE necessitate continuation of oral anticoagulation. Closure with an endocardial or epicardial device could be attempted. Depending on the size and morphology of the gap, the closure device could range from an atrial septal occluder, vascular plug, to a LAA occluder. An endovascular device may not be suitable for crescent-shaped gaps; epicardial ligation could be performed. However, adhesions from previous pericardial access may prevent further attempts. Similarly a septal occluder can be used to close incomplete closures following an epicardial approach. To ensure complete closure and to prevent device embolization, attention to sizing and follow-up TEE are essential.

Device Dislodgment and Embolism

Judicious attention to device sizing and the pre-release criteria reduces the risk of dislodgment and embolism. In the event a device may require recapturing, a transseptal or transaortic approach may be attempted depending on the location of the device. A snare or bioptome can be used to capture the device. Another important consideration is the retrievable method; predetermining the preclosure method and sheath size ensure the device can be removed.

SUMMARY

Endovascular closure and epicardial ligation of the LAA are clinically feasible alternatives to oral anticoagulation for nonvalvular AF. The procedure on the whole is intuitive; however, because no appendages are the same, there are tips and tricks that will reduce the learning curve and improve procedural results.

REFERENCES

1. Reddy VY, Doshi SK, Sievert H, et al, PROTECT AF Investigators. Percutaneous left atrial appendage closure for stroke prophylaxis in patients with atrial fibrillation: 2.3-year follow-up of the PROTECT AF (Watchman Left Atrial Appendage System for embolic protection in patients with atrial fibrillation) trial. Circulation 2013;127:720–9.
2. Wang Y, Di Biase L, Horton RP, et al. Left atrial appendage studied by computed tomography to help planning for appendage closure device placement. J Cardiovasc Electrophysiol 2010;21:973–82.
3. AGA Medical Corporation. AMPLATZER cardiac plug clinical trial. Bethesda (MD): National Library of Medicine (US); 2000. Available at: http://clinicaltrials.gov/show/NCT01118299. NLM Identifier: NCT01118299. Accessed July 1, 2013.
4. Franzen O, Reddy V, Worthley S, et al. Clinical experience with the Coherex WAVECREST left atrial appendage occlusion system: acute results from the WAVECREST I trial. EuroPCR 2013 Congress. Paris, France, May 23, 2013.
5. Bagai J, Zhao D. Subcutaneous "Figure-of-Eight" stitch to achieve hemostasis after removal of large-caliber femoral venous sheaths. Cardiac Interv Today 2008;5:22–3.

Role of Transesophageal Echocardiography in Left Atrial Appendage Device Closure

David M. Dudzinski, MD, JD[a,b],
Shmuel Schwartzenberg, MD[a,b],
Gaurav A. Upadhyay, MD[a,c], Judy Hung, MD[a,b],*

KEYWORDS

- Left atrial appendage • Percutaneously implanted devices • Transesophageal echocardiography

KEY POINTS

- Left atrial appendage (LAA) occlusion or ligation by percutaneously implanted devices is increasingly an alternative management option for atrial fibrillation, particularly for patients who are intolerant of or have contraindications for anticoagulation.
- Echocardiography plays an important part in screening, guidance of implantation, and after-device assessment.
- Important functions of echocardiography include assessment of LAA anatomy suitable for device implantation, thrombus exclusion, guidance of transseptal puncture, localization of catheter, guidance of device deployment, and after-device assessment.

INTRODUCTION

Left atrial appendage (LAA) occlusion or ligation by percutaneously implanted devices is increasingly an alternative management option for atrial fibrillation, particularly for patients who are intolerant or have contraindications for anticoagulation. Echocardiography plays an important part in screening, guidance of implantation, and after-device assessment. Assessment of LAA anatomy suitable for device implantation, thrombus exclusion, guidance of transseptal puncture, localization of catheter, guidance of device deployment, and after-device assessment are all important functions of echocardiography. This article reviews the role of echocardiography in device-based LAA occlusion or ligation.

LAA ANATOMY

The LAA is a blind-end tubular pouch of variable geometry that is an embryologic remnant of the primitive left atrium. The functions of this appendage have not yet been robustly defined, but theories suggest it could play roles in mediation of thirst, in endocrine signaling, and in fluid and sodium homeostasis by producing atrial natriuretic peptide and offloading an overloaded left atrium because of relatively higher distensibility.[1] Its clinical importance stems from being the nidus of clot location in cardioembolic syndromes.

The LAA has been described as tubular in shape but in reality exhibits rather heterogenous anatomy across the population. Only about 20% of patients at autopsy have a single-lobed and tubular structure, with more than half of patients having a bilobed structure and about one-quarter of patients having 3 or more lobes.[2] More recent studies have used multimodality cardiac imaging techniques to define in vivo subtypes of LAA shape.[3] In a recent cardiac computed tomographic and magnetic resonance study of 932 consecutive

The authors have nothing to disclose.
[a] Cardiology Division, Massachusetts General Hospital, 55 Fruit Street, Boston, MA 02114, USA;
[b] Echocardiography Laboratory, Massachusetts General Hospital, 55 Fruit Street, Boston, MA 02114, USA;
[c] Cardiac Electrophysiology Division, Massachusetts General Hospital, 55 Fruit Street, Boston, MA 02114, USA
* Corresponding author.
E-mail address: jhung@partners.org

Intervent Cardiol Clin 3 (2014) 255–280
http://dx.doi.org/10.1016/j.iccl.2013.12.005
2211-7458/14/$ – see front matter © 2014 Elsevier Inc. All rights reserved.

patients with drug-refractory atrial fibrillation referred for ablation, 4 primary anatomic shapes were defined (**Fig. 1**, **Table 1**).

The chicken-wing morphology (see **Fig. 1**A) consists of a central tubular structure that displays a clear bend at the base of the appendage after the atrial-appendage anastomosis. The cactus morphology has a central lobe with multiple accessory lobes extending superiorly and inferiorly. Windsock morphology, like chicken-wing, has a dominant central lobe but may also have several secondary and tertiary lobes that are oriented in directions different than cactus morphology and unlike chicken-wing lacks the characteristic bend. The cauliflower morphology is irregular with multiple side lobes arising from a relatively short central lobe in contrast to chicken-wing and windsock shapes. These morphologies robustly correlated with risk of prior transient ischemic attack (TIA)/stroke (CVA) in the 932 patient cohort, with a 3-fold higher prevalence in the non-chicken-wing morphologies relative to chicken-wing morphology based on multivariate analysis (odds ratio 2.95, $P = .041$). Among the patients in the cohort with a CHADS2 score of 0 to 1, prior TIA/stroke was 10-fold more prevalent in the non-chicken-wing morphologies after multivariate analysis (odds ratio 10.1, $P = .019$).

The internal lateral wall of the LAA is trabeculated with pectinate muscle fibers that are oriented in parallel. The pectinate muscles are important because echocardiographically they must be distinguished from thrombi. Pectinate muscles measure more than 1 mm in thickness in 97% of patients, with thinner pectinate muscles observed only in the first and last decades of life.[2] Between the pectinate muscles, the wall of the appendage is extremely thin.[4] It has been observed in atrial fibrillation patients that the wall is smoother (which may possibly correlate with increased appendage volume).[4] The portion of the appendage harboring pectinate muscles is an embryologic remnant of the primitive left atrium, while the smoother-walled remainder derives from primordial pulmonary vein tissue.[1,5]

The LAA arises from the anterolateral aspect of the left atrium along the atrioventricular groove between the mitral valve and the left pulmonary vein apertures, and in general, projects anteriorly; the exact vector and anatomy depend on specific LAA morphology, as some appendages project inferiorly, posteriorly, or superiorly.[4] The

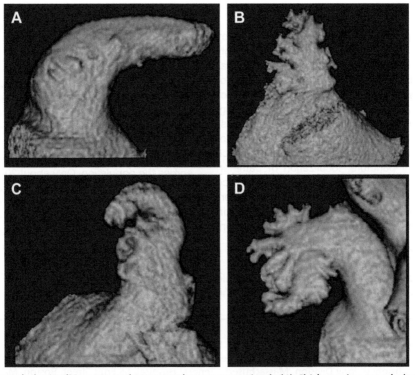

Fig. 1. LAA morphologies (3D computed tomography reconstructions). (*A*) Chicken-wing morphology. (*B*) Cactus morphology. (*C*) Windsock morphology. (*D*) Cauliflower morphology. (*From* Di Biase L, Santangeli P, Anselmino M, et al. Does the left atrial appendage morphology correlate with the risk of stroke in patients with atrial fibrillation? J Am Coll Cardiol 2012;60:533–4; with permission.)

Table 1
Left atrial appendage morphologies

Morphology	Prevalence of Morphology (%)	Patients in Cohort with Stroke/TIA (%)	Odds Ratio CVA/TIA vs Chicken Wing
Chicken wing	48	4	n/a
Cactus	30	12	4.08, P = .046
Windsock	19	10	4.8, P = .38
Cauliflower	3	18	8.02, P = .056

Data from Di Biase L, Santangeli P, Anselmino M, et al. Does the left atrial appendage morphology correlate with the risk of stroke in patients with atrial fibrillation? J Am Coll Cardiol 2012;60:531–8.

atrioventricular groove separates the appendage from the left ventricle, and the left circumflex artery (and great cardiac vein) can be visualized in both pathologic and echocardiographic cross-section in the atrioventricular groove. The left superior pulmonary vein anastomosis with the left atrium is posterosuperior to and abuts the left atrium-LAA anastomosis. These anastomoses are separated by a fibrous ridge of atrial myocardium that is referred to as the "left lateral ridge"[4] or colloquially as "coumadin ridge," (**Fig. 2**) owing to possible early echocardiographic mischaracterization of this structure as thrombus or atrial mass.[6] Within this muscular ridge runs remnants of the vein of Marshall, some nerve issue, and arteries, which in some patients may supply the sinus node.

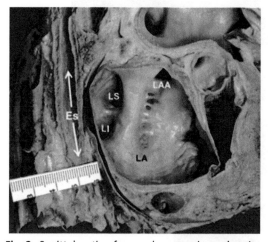

Fig. 2. Sagittal section from cadaver specimen showing the relationship of the left atrial appendage (LAA)-left atrial junction in close proximity to the left superior (LS) and left inferior (LI) pulmonary vein apertures, which are separated by a band of tissue (left lateral ridge or "coumadin ridge"). Es, esophagus; LA, left atrium. (*From* Calkins H, Ho SY, Cabrera JA, et al. Anatomy of the left atrium and pulmonary veins. In: Natale A, Raviele A, editors. Atrial fibrillation ablation: the state of the art based on the Venice chart International Consensus Document. New York: Wiley-Blackwell; 2007; with permission.)

The atrial-appendage junction or orifice is not perfectly round but rather ovoid. Even in a multi-lobed appendage, the appendage base is often tubular and thus the orifice of the left atrium-LAA junction remains ellipsoid in cross-section. Approximate dimensions based on analysis of gross specimens show a mean major diameter of 17.4 mm and a mean minor diameter of 10.9 mm, with the plane of the orifice oriented obliquely to the mitral annular plane.[7] Some data suggest that higher burden of chronic atrial fibrillation is correlated with increasing orifice size and a more round shape.[8]

The LAA neighbors in the anteroposterior dimension are generally the left superior pulmonary vein posteriorly and main/left pulmonary artery trunk anteriorly[4]; the lung lies to the left and the left ventricle proper to the right, while the pulmonary artery provides part of the superior border and left ventricle provides the inferior border. The pulmonary vasculature neighbors help define pericardial abutments to the appendage, with the left pulmonic vein recess of the pericardium forming part of the posterior border, and the transverse sinus, specifically the left pulmonic recess, forming parts of the superior, anterior, and inferior border (**Fig. 3**).[9] Because of the close approximation of the left ventricle and appendage with both structures constrained by the pericardium, left ventricular function and dilation in diastole may be key determinants of LAA outflow.

ECHOCARDIOGRAPHIC EXAMINATION OF THE LAA

The LAA is typically visible only on transesophageal echocardiography (TEE) due to its posterior position in the far-field from the transthoracic transducer. Accordingly, TEE is used for reliable procedural guidance when visualization of the appendage is necessary. Nevertheless, in certain patients the LAA is visible on transthoracic echocardiography in basal short-axis or in apical views, depending on the appendage size, geometry, and relation to other cardiac structures (**Fig. 4**).

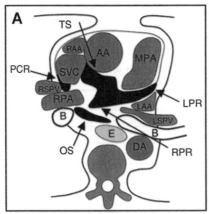 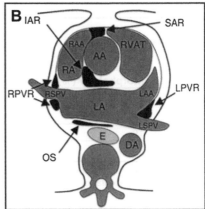

Fig. 3. (*A*) Schematic of cross-section of cardiac anatomy at the level of the right pulmonary artery (RPA). The left pulmonic recess, a part of the transverse sinus, lies between the main pulmonary artery (MPA) and left atrial appendage (LAA). (*B*) Schematic of cross-section of cardiac anatomy below the level of the right pulmonary artery. The left pulmonic vein recess is a potential space between the LAA and the left superior pulmonic vein. AA, ascending aorta; B, bronchi; DA, descending aorta; E, esophagus; IAR, inferior aortic recess; LA, left atrium; LPR, left pulmonic recess; LPVR, left pulmonic vein recess; LSPV, left superior pulmonary vein; OS, oblique sinus; PCR, postcaval recess; RA, right atrium; RAA, right atrial appendage; RPR, right pulmonic recess; RPVR, right pulmonic vein recess; RSPV, right superior pulmonary vein; RVAT, right ventricular outflow tract; SAR, superior aortic recess; SVC, superior vena cava; TS, transverse sinus. (*From* Groell R, Schlaffer GJ, Rienmueller R. Pericardial sinuses and recesses: findings at electrocardiographically triggered electron-beam CT. Radiology 1999;212:70–1; with permission.)

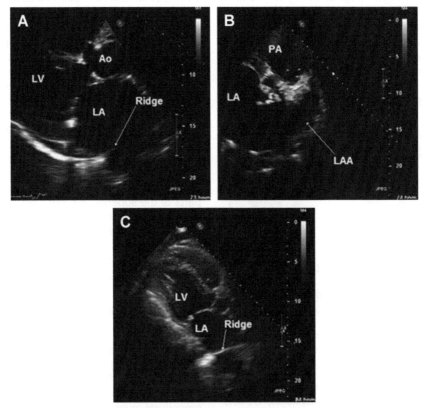

Fig. 4. (*A, B*) TTE of a 78-year-old man with morbid obesity, hypertension, and atrial fibrillation admitted with marked volume overload. Dilated left ventricle and left atrium are visible, as well as the coumadin ridge on (*A*) taken from the parasternal long-axis view, and in (*B*) in the short-axis view, the appendage with tip projecting anteriorly toward the pulmonary artery. (*C*) Coumadin ridge on a TTE image from parasternal long-axis view on a 63-year-old man admitted with fever, respiratory distress, and murmur. Ao, aorta; LA, left atrium; LAA, left atrial appendage; LPV, left-sided pulmonary vein; LV, left ventricle; PA, pulmonary artery.

The comprehensive transesophageal examination of the LAA requires careful attention and interrogation in multiple views, planes, and angulations to ensure that any and all accessory lobes are identified and possible thrombi are detected and distinguished from normal pectinate muscle anatomy.[10] In addition to 2-dimensional (2D) imaging, the complete echocardiographic examination includes both color Doppler and pulse wave Doppler as a collateral assessment of thrombi. Three-dimensional (3D) imaging can also improve the accuracy in distinguishing pectinate muscles versus thrombi.[11]

The appendage is routinely visible from the midesophageal station with 2 cardinal views that show the appendage: the basal short-axis view where the appendage is juxtaposed to the aortic valve (typically at lower omniplane angles), and a 2-chamber view where the relationships of the appendage to the left atrium and left ventricle are manifest (typically at higher omniplane angles) (Fig. 5).[12] Omniplane capability allows visualization of the appendage through the entire range of possible angles, often from 0° to 150°, and each of these views provides information and may reveal accessory lobes not seen in other views (Fig. 6). At the lower omniplane angles (0–50°), the probe must be rotated left (counterclockwise) to bring the appendage into view; conversely, at higher omniplane angles (>80–100°), the probe may need to be rotated right (clockwise). In all windows, the probe may need to be withdrawn (eg, moved more cephalad in the esophagus) or advanced to keep the appendage in view.

A thorough examination such as in Fig. 6 will provide clues as to whether there are multiple lobes or accessory lobes. Fig. 7 shows how the appendage may appear to have no accessory lobes until a view with a high omniplane angle view is achieved. Bilobed appendages are shown in Fig. 8 and a multilobed appendage is shown in Fig. 9. Simultaneous biplane (or X-plane) imaging is useful to identify appendages with occult accessory lobes (Fig. 10).

Echocardiography helps characterize the internal ultrastructure of the appendage and differentiates the findings from thrombus. Occasionally muscular ridges in the appendage (Fig. 11) will divide accessory lobes from the main body and these ridges must be distinguished from thrombi. The pectinate muscles are one of the dominant features of the appendage anatomy. Typically 1- to 2-mm-thick, the pectinate muscles can exhibit a wide variety of echocardiographic appearances (Figs. 12 and 13).

The primary anatomic neighbors of the LAA that are readily visible at echocardiography include the left superior pulmonary vein (Fig. 14), left lateral ridge (Figs. 15 and 16), atrioventricular groove vessels (Fig. 17), and the pericardial space (Fig. 18). It is essential to distinguish the left superior pulmonary vein from the appendage because

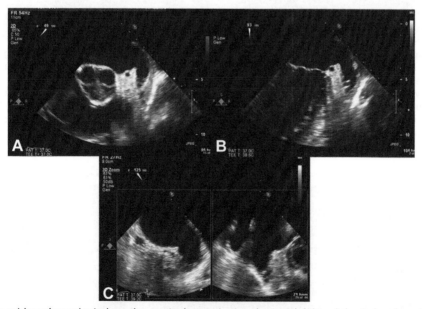

Fig. 5. In the midesophageal window, the aortic short-axis view (~0–50°) (A) and the 2-chamber view with the left atrium and left ventricle (80°–120°) (B) each show the appendage. X-plane imaging can be used to simultaneously assess the appendage in both of these views (C). In panels A, B, and the left side of panel C, the left coronary artery is visible in cross-section.

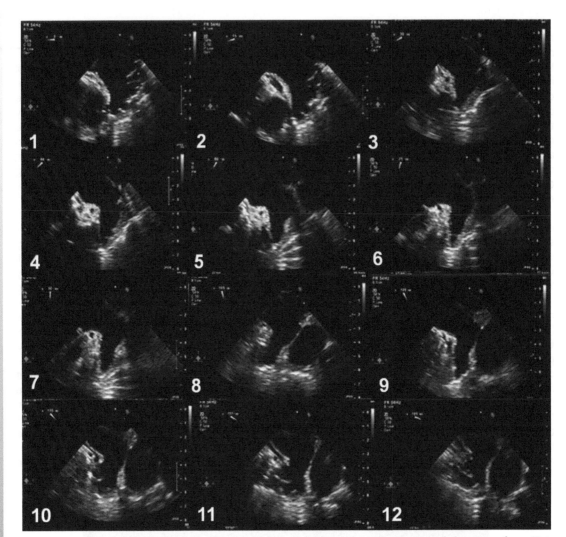

Fig. 6. Omniplane imaging allows visualization of the appendage throughout most of the range from 0° to almost 180°. Panel starts from 0° on the omniplane, increasing approximately 15° on the omniplane with each successive panel. This level of detail helps the echocardiographer to construct a mental 3D map of the appendage, which is useful to identify accessory lobes, assess the atrial-appendage orifice, and robustly evaluate pectinate muscles and exclude thrombus. At lower omniplane angles the echocardiographer may have to turn the probe to the left (counterclockwise) to maintain the appendage in view, whereas rightward (clockwise) rotation will be required at higher omniplane angles.

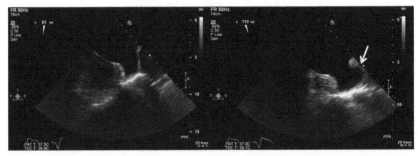

Fig. 7. Up to an omniplane angle of 100° (*left panel*), the appendage appeared to be tubular without an accessory lobe; at 110° (*right panel*), an accessory lobe was visualized (toward 2 o'clock, *white arrow*).

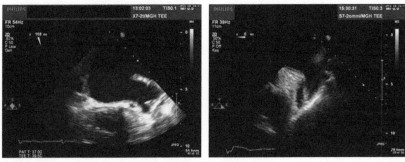

Fig. 8. Bilobed LAAs shown at 0° (*left panel*) and 110° (*right panel*).

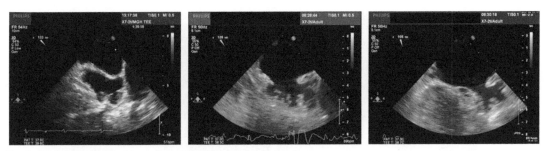

Fig. 9. Multilobed LAAs (shown at 100°–110° on omniplane).

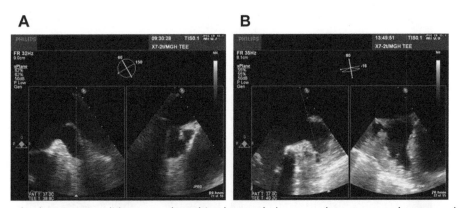

Fig. 10. Single-plane imaging did not reveal anything but a tubular appendage structure; however, addition of an orthogonal plane with X-plane shows accessory lobes in each of these 2 examples (pointing toward 1 o'clock in right part of *panel A*, and toward 9 o'clock in right part of *panel B*).

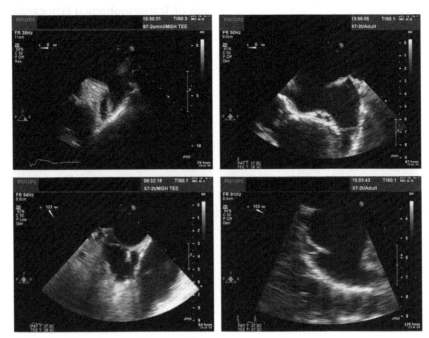

Fig. 11. Examples of muscular ridges in the LAA cavity.

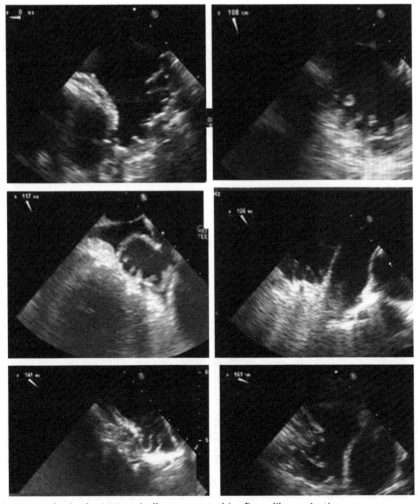

Fig. 12. Pectinate muscles in the LAA typically appear as thin, fingerlike projections.

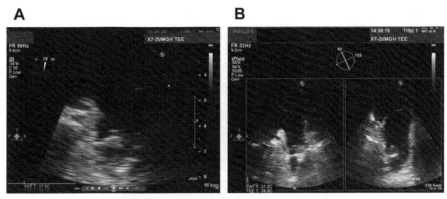

Fig. 13. (A, B) Thickened pectinate muscles need to be distinguished from thrombi.

in patients with atypical anatomy this vein may be mistaken for the appendage cavity. In patients with a small pericardial fluid collection in the transverse sinus, the echolucent space may be mistaken for the appendage; pericardial space can generally be distinguished from the appendage by an inability to document a communication with the atrium proper (as well as by color and spectral Doppler).

Assessment of the appendage orifice is necessary in guiding approaches to the appendage apex. Although the opening can be assessed in multiple planes (eg, see **Fig. 6**), 3D echocardiography affords en-face views of the total area of the orifice (**Fig. 19**).

Spontaneous echo contrast (SEC) represents the macroscopically visible agglomeration of erythrocytes into a rouleaux formation in the setting of stagnant flow (**Fig. 20**). High echocardiographic gain settings may overestimate SEC. In part based on gain settings and the ambient degree of SEC, a qualitative scale of 1 to 4 from mild, transiently detectable SEC on high gain settings to very intense and readily detectable SEC can be used to grade degrees of SEC.[12] SEC correlates with rates of thromboembolism, including a 4% to 5% rate of stroke despite therapy with aspirin and therapeutic warfarin.[13] SEC that is more organized becomes "sludge" or highly viscous and adherent blood (**Fig. 21**). Both SEC and sludge are thought

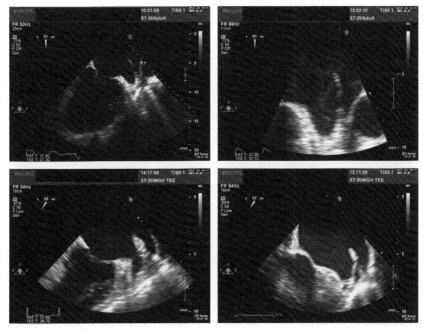

Fig. 14. These views in the midesophageal 2-chamber window show the relationship of the appendage to the left superior pulmonary vein and the pulmonary artery.

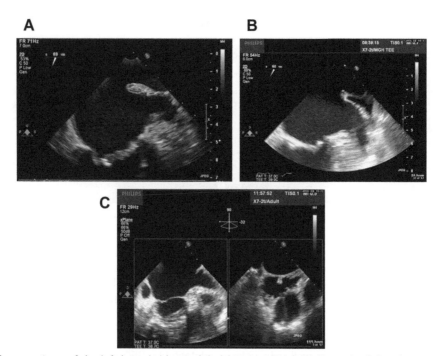

Fig. 15. Close-up views of the left lateral ridge in (*A*). (*B*) Pericardial fluid (from the left pulmonic vein recess) outlining the space between the left superior pulmonary vein and the left lateral ridge. (*C*) A biplane view of the ridge that shows the muscular tissue protruding from the ridge inferiorly toward the appendage orifice (eg, pointing toward 6 o'clock in the right panel).

to represent intermediate states on the continuum of stasis and coagulation to overt thrombus (**Fig. 22**). Sludge and clot both manifest as filling defects with color Doppler or contrast, if used. Clots need to be distinguished from artifacts due to acoustic shadowing from the warfarin ridge as well as parts of the appendage wall (**Fig. 23**).

DOPPLER CHARACTERISTICS OF LAA FUNCTION

The temporal characteristics of contractile function of the appendage are similar to that of the atrium, although the contraction pattern is distinct with appendage contraction primarily at the apex resulting in obliteration of the cavity (the base contributes relatively little to the appendage contraction).[5] The appendage exhibits Doppler flow patterns that are distinct from that of the left atrium proper and that are dependent on the ambient atrial rhythm. On the transesophageal color Doppler examination, LAA outflows will be orange and inflows will be blue (**Fig. 24**). In appendages with low inflow and outflow velocities, the Nyquist limits should be decreased to best ascertain the flow velocity. Color Doppler can be

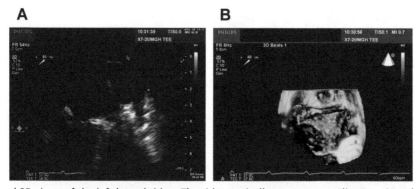

Fig. 16. 2D and 3D views of the left lateral ridge. The ridge typically appears as a "line" on 2D echo (*A*), but 3D echo (*B*) better shows that it is a structure running along the left atrium wall and separating the left superior and left inferior pulmonary veins from the appendage orifice.

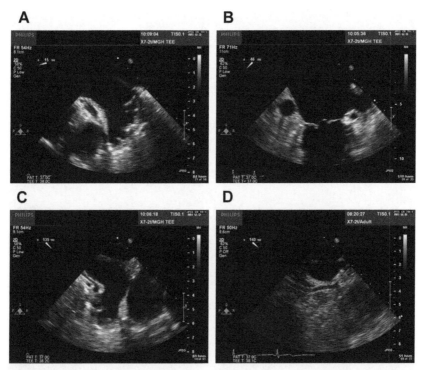

Fig. 17. Left coronary artery branches running in the atrioventricular groove as juxtaposed to the appendage. (*A, C*) From the same patient, the left coronary artery is seen in cross-section at 15° and along the longitudinal axis at 135°. (*B*) Taken at 46°, the left circumflex in the atrioventricular groove on the right of the mitral annulus, with the coronary sinus at the left of the mitral annulus. (*D*) Taken at 140° is another longitudinal view of the circumflex artery. See **Fig. 5** for other examples of left coronary artery anatomy.

used to discern whether an echodensity is an artifact, as in **Fig. 25**.

For the Doppler pulse wave examination, the cursor is typically placed about 1 cm into the appendage neck[14] (as opposed to at the atrial-appendage junction), while avoiding artifacts from wall motion as the appendage tapers toward its apex.[10] However, cursor location has not been standardized formally[12]; some recommend

sampling at a location that maximizes visual color Doppler flow. The Doppler examination should always be performed in at least 2 different appendage views.

The appendage function and the corresponding Doppler flows vary with rhythm. Based on ambient atrial rhythm, 4 types of appendage Doppler velocity profiles have been established: type I, sinus rhythm; type II, atrial flutter; type III, atrial fibrillation

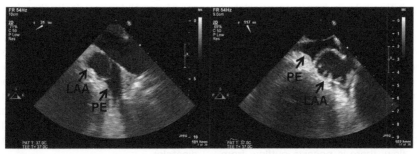

Fig. 18. Pericardial fluid surrounding the appendage. On these views, the pericardial recess could be mistaken for the appendage cavity unless the echocardiographer works through multiple planes to show that the atrium is not connected to this space and/or applies color and pulse wave Doppler modes, important because fibrin strands or debris in the pericardial space may be confused with appendage thrombus. LAA, left atrial appendage; PE, pericardial effusion.

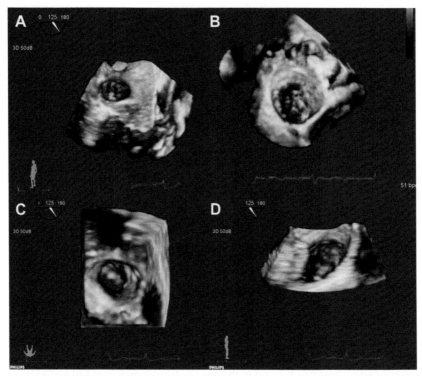

Fig. 19. The appendage orifice appears ovoid on 3D views (*A* and *C*). (*B*) A picture of (*A*) rotated to bring the mitral annulus into cross-sectional view and reveals a cut-away view of the proximal appendage. (*D*) A picture of (*C*) that was rotated 90° clockwise, then 90° cephalad, and then cut away to reveal the appendage in cross-section.

(with velocities >20 cm/s); type IV, atrial fibrillation (with velocities ≤20 cm/s).

In sinus rhythm, the Doppler waveform displays 4 characteristic phases: appendage contraction, appendage filling, systolic reflection waves, and early diastolic outflow (**Fig. 26**).[10] Like the atrium proper, the LAA in sinus rhythm contracts after the P wave on the electrocardiogram; this contraction produces a relatively high-velocity outflow (60 ± 14 cm/s) on the Doppler tracing, which is analogous to and simultaneous with the mitral A wave.[5] This velocity has been correlated with appendage contractile function. Atrial and LAA diastole occurs after the mitral valve has closed and the QRS complex appears; this filling, while not mechanistically fully characterized, results in a negative velocity on the Doppler profile (52 ± 13 cm/s). During ventricular systole there may be passive bidirectional outflows and inflows manifesting as reflections of the contraction and filling waves. Shortly after early passive atrial-to-ventricular flow, there is passive outflow from the appendage to the atrium proper, akin to the mitral E wave; the mechanism is compression from the filled left ventricle and suction from the emptied left atrium. Throughout ventricular

diastole up until appendage contraction, there may be low-velocity continuous inflow, in part from pulmonary veins.

In atrial flutter there is regular atrial activity and the appendage Doppler waveform mimics the electrocardiographic morphology with regularly alternating high-velocity peaks (**Fig. 27**). Although the LAA may still contract in atrial fibrillation, typically the appendage waveform in atrial fibrillation is characterized by irregularly alternating positive and negative peaks with varying amplitudes that are of overall lower velocity than in sinus rhythm or atrial flutter (**Fig. 28**).[12,15] The higher atrial contraction rate in atrial fibrillation as compared with atrial flutter implies that each contraction involves a lesser volume of blood and this may partly explain why average velocities are lower. In both atrial fibrillation and atrial flutter, and in certain types of pacing, the velocities seen when the mitral valve is closed (eg, ventricular systole) are lower than when the mitral valve is open (ventricular diastole).

Combinations of color and spectral Doppler imaging can help to distinguish the appendage from other neighboring structures; **Fig. 29** shows that the structure thought on 2D imaging to be the

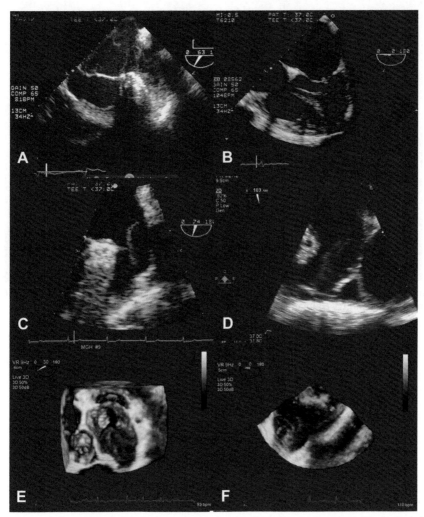

Fig. 20. SEC is seen as echodense accumulations of red blood cells. (*A*) Extensive SEC in both the left atrium and the appendage. (*B*) SEC in the left atrium proper. (*C, D*) More organized SEC in the LAA. (*E*) 3D pictures of SEC filling the appendage, which is seen protruding into the atrium body in (*F*).

appendage was in fact the left superior pulmonary vein.

The peak left atrium outflow velocity is a proxy of left atrial appendage contractile function and this measure is an important predictor of thromboembolic events, including in patients in sinus rhythm.[16] Peak outflow velocities are averaged over 3 cardiac cycles in sinus rhythm, to up to 10

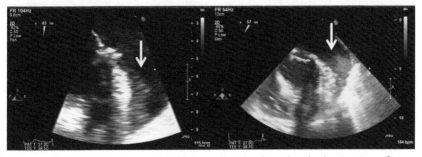

Fig. 21. Sludge is blood that is nearly organized into a discrete thrombus by lamination of stagnant layers of blood *in situ* (*arrows*).

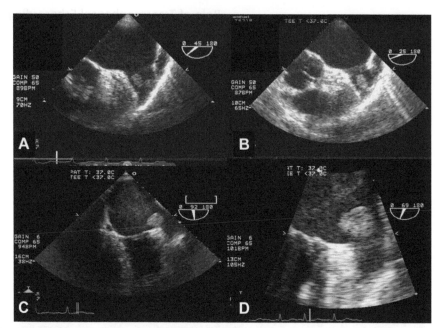

Fig. 22. Examples of thrombi in the LAA. Thrombi are well-circumscribed mobile echodensities. (*A*, *B*) Images from the same patient, and (*C*, *D*) images from the same patient.

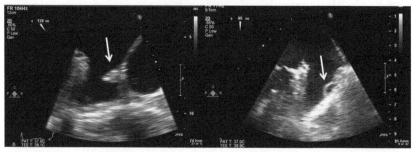

Fig. 23. Left panel shows an echodensity (*arrow*) that is a muscular part of the appendage wall. Right panel shows invagination of the wall (*arrow*) due to fluid in the pericardial space.

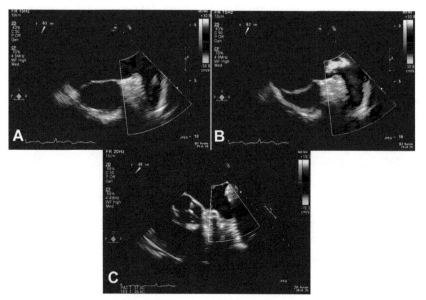

Fig. 24. Color Doppler analysis of inflow (*A*) and outflow (*B*) into an appendage with vigorous flow. (*C*) Note that the Nyquist limits are decreased in an attempt to detect signal in an appendage with stagnant flow.

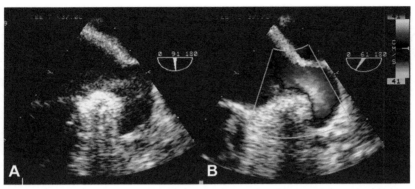

Fig. 25. Color Doppler confirms that the echodensity in the proximal LAA (*A*) is an artifact, because if the echodensity was sludge or clot, it would manifest as a filling defect on the color Doppler (*B*).

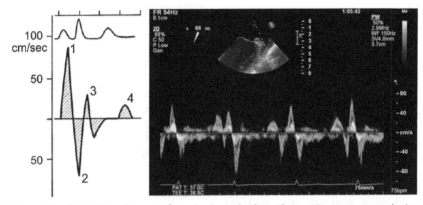

Fig. 26. Left, Schematic of LAA Doppler waveform in sinus rhythm. The y-axis represents velocity of flow, with positive velocities indicating outflow from the appendage and negative velocities inflows. Deflection 1 is LAA contraction that occurs in late diastole and generally has the highest amplitude. Deflection 2 represents filling of the atrial appendage that occurs in early ventricular systole. Deflection 3 represents systolic reflection waves; variable multiples of reflections of waves 1 and 2 may occur. Deflection 4 represents early diastolic passive emptying of the appendage. Right, A representative tracing of LAA Doppler velocity profile in sinus rhythm. (*[Left] From* Agmon Y, Khandheria BK, Gentile F, et al. Echocardiographic assessment of the left atrial appendage. J Am Coll Cardiol 1999;34:1867–77; with permission.)

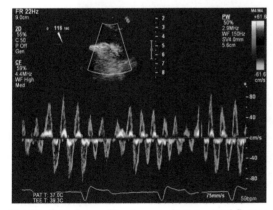

Fig. 27. Doppler profile of appendage in atrial flutter. Note the overall lower velocities during ventricular systole compared with ventricular diastole.

cardiac cycles in atrial fibrillation.[12,14,15] The Stroke Prevention in Atrial Fibrillation III trial showed that peak outflow velocity of less than 20 cm/s correlated significantly with the presence of dense SEC, appendage thrombus, and cardioembolic events.[15] Mean peak outflow velocity obtained on TEE at the time of cardioversion predicts both success of cardioversion (>31 cm/s, OR 2.8 of success, $P = .0013$)[17] and also the likelihood of maintaining sinus rhythm for up to 1 year (>40 cm/s, OR 5.2, $P = .0001$).[14]

Besides rhythm, other contributors to the appendage velocities include age, gender, heart rate, volume status, left ventricle function, and mitral valve disease. Peak velocities of outflow and inflow appear to decrease with increasing age.[18,19]

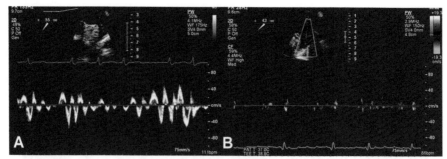

Fig. 28. (*A, B*) Doppler flow tracings from the LAA in two different patients in atrial fibrillation, both taken on the same velocity scale. Panel A shows average peak velocities >20 cm/s, whereas panel B shows average peak velocities <20 cm/s. Mean peak flows <20 cm/s correlate with higher thromboembolic risk.

PERIPROCEDURAL GUIDANCE IN LAA PROCEDURES

Transseptal Puncture

Deployment of devices requires access to the left atrium body, which is conventionally obtained via a transseptal approach. The interatrial septum is a more complex 3D structure than a simple plane separating the right and left atria.[4,20] A rim of infolded atrial muscular issue surrounds the fossa ovalis, and the transseptal puncture is typically targeted to the fossa ovalis given this location represents a minimal transseptal thickness.[20] The specific orientation of the transseptal plane depends on ventricular geometry as well as thoracic and skeletal anatomy (eg, may be altered in emphysema, kyphosis).[4] As about

one-quarter of the population has a patent communication via the fossa ovalis, this can be a viable target site for transseptal crossing under TEE guidance.

The interatrial septum is accessed from wires and devices placed via a peripheral venotomy and then maneuvered to the right atrium. On 2D TEE, septal puncture is monitored on interatrial septum views, typically at done from midesophageal window with omniplane angles at either 40° to 60° and/or 90° to 120° (**Fig. 30**A–C). 2D techniques display the interatrial septum in cross-sectional planes.[20] On these planes the relatively thicker muscular rim surrounding the fossa ovalis is visualized as a linear structure, and the overall view with fossa ovalis between en-face views of

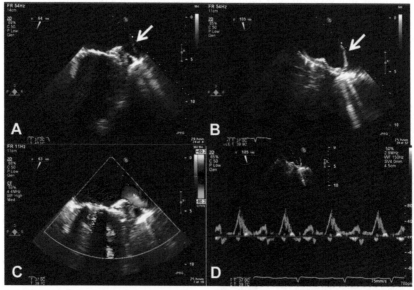

Fig. 29. Panels A and B show what appears to be the LAA (*arrows*). However, color (*C*) and Doppler profile (*D*) confirm that the structure is a pulmonary vein, because there was no inflow (a *blue jet*) seen and there is a characteristic pulmonary vein Doppler signature. Subsequent to the TEE, records were obtained that confirmed the patient had had a previous surgical ligation of the appendage.

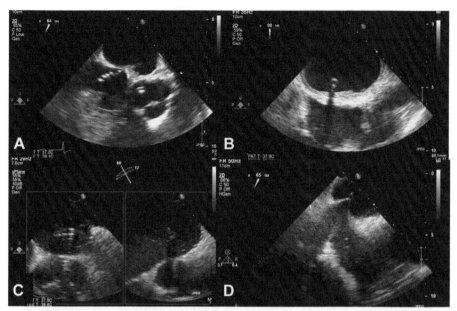

Fig. 30. (*A*) The catheter approaching the interatrial septum in a 60-degree view, and (*B*) shows the approach in the bicaval view. (*C*) X-plane imaging used to monitor both views simultaneously. (*D*) "Tenting" of the interatrial septum.

a thicker muscular rim is sometimes referred to as having a "dumbbell" shape, especially prominent in cases of fatty infiltration of the interatrial septum.[4,20] On 2D views, the wire from the right atrium can be visualized to "tent" and then perforate the fossa ovalis (see **Fig. 30**D). The 2D imaging plane will have to be adjusted to ensure the catheter remains in the plane of the ultrasound so as to guide it from left atrium to the appendage (**Fig. 31**). Sometimes the patent foramen ovale can be used as the site of puncture, and echocardiography will help define the anatomy and orientation of the foramen tunnel for use as transseptal crossing.

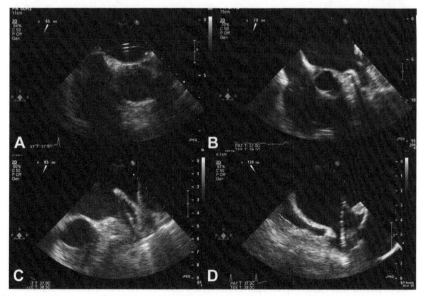

Fig. 31. Guiding the catheter to the LAA. (*A, B*) Different omniplane views are required to visualize the catheter within the left atrium body. (*C, D*) Different omniplane angles can be used to confirm positioning of a catheter in the apex of the appendage.

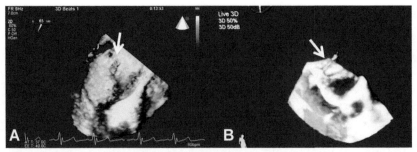

Fig. 32. 3D views of the interatrial septum provide additional information in targeting the approach in transseptal puncture. (*A, B*) Interatrial septum as viewed from the left atrium showing the location of the transeptal puncture (*arrows*). Panel B is angled more superiorly.

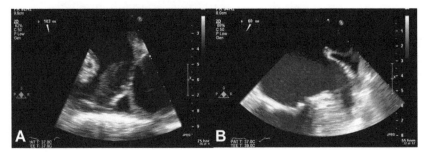

Fig. 33. Effusions surrounding the LAA in the transverse sinus between the appendage and pulmonary artery (*A*) and the left pulmonic vein recess (*B*).

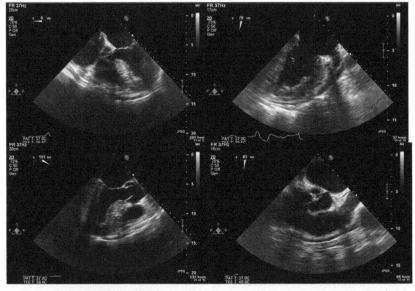

Fig. 34. TEE views of pericardial fluid. Top left panel shows a 4-chamber view with pericardial fluid anterior to the right ventricle. Top right shows a 2-chamber view and bottom left panel shows a 3-chamber view, each with pericardial fluid anterior to the left ventricle. Bottom right panel is a short-axis view at the level of the aortic valve, which reveals fluid anterior to the right ventricle.

Table 2	
Visualization of pericardial effusion at TEE	
Echocardiographic View	**Pericardial Effusion Location**
Midesophageal, 4 chamber	RV free wall, LV lateral wall
Midesophageal, 2 chamber	LV anterior and inferior walls
Midesophageal, aortic long axis	Transverse sinus
Midesophageal, aortic short axis	Anterior RV base/free wall
Transgastric, short axis	Circumferential LV, circumferential RV
Transgastric, long axis	RV free wall, LV anterior and inferior walls

3D echocardiography is increasingly being used for real-time procedural guidance given augmented definition of the nuances of the septum anatomy with an "en-face" view, as well as identification of neighboring structures (**Fig. 32**).[20] 3D echocardiography may be especially useful in patients with unusual anatomy of the interatrial septum (eg, aneurysm), rotation of the cardiac axis due to cardiac or extracardiac chest

pathologic abnormality, or those who are undergoing repeat transseptal puncture. Although the 3D acquisition will engender lower the frame rates, operators have reported that this is not a particular problem in most patients because the septum is generally relatively immobile (excepting cases of septal aneurysm) and the catheter also remains relatively fixed at the point of transseptal puncture.[20]

Localization of the Catheter in the LAA

The appendage orifice is an ovoid structure with a major dimension of about 1.7 cm on average and thus a total orifice area of about 1.5 cm². 2D and 3D echocardiography are useful to guide the catheter to the appendage orifice after transseptal puncture. After puncture, on 2D echocardiography the omniplane angle will have to be continually adjusted to keep the catheter in the imaging plane (see **Fig. 31**). As above, the atrial-appendage junction is oblique rather than perfectly perpendicular relative to the mitral annulus. Guidance is also useful in approaching the appendage given that the left pulmonic veins and branches of the left coronary artery all run within 10 mm of the orifice. Moreover, in approximately 30% of the population the sinus artery node travels in the left lateral ridge, and external to the appendage in the pericardial

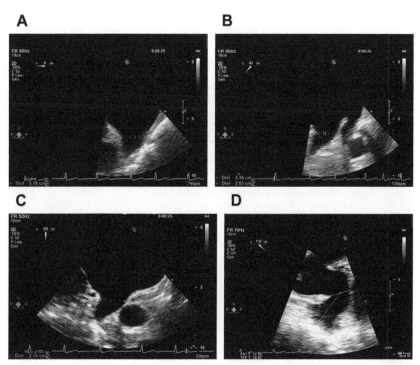

Fig. 35. (*A*) LAA at 0° TEE omniplane. (*B*) LAA at 45° TEE omniplane. (*C*) LAA at 90° TEE omniplane. (*D*) LAA at 135° TEE omniplane.

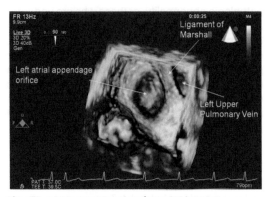

Fig. 36. LAA reconstruction from 3D images.

space the left phrenic nerve is found. There may also be significant lymphatic channels. These peri-orifice structures are in jeopardy when devices for appendage deployment are oversized, which is a necessary consideration when trying to fit a round device in an oval-shaped hole. Correct sizing of LAA closure devices can help prevent both trauma due to oversizing and incomplete closure from oversizing. 3D TEE with en-face viewing of the appendage orifice[21] improves accuracy of sizing compared with 2D echocardiography (with computed tomography as reference) and positioning; 2D echocardiography more often results in undersizing.[8] Echocardiography with color and Doppler modes also helps confirm complete exclusion of the appendage from the atrium proper, which is crucial because residual shunts

may predispose to thrombus due to impaired flows in the appendage.[21]

Assessment of Pericardial Effusion on Echocardiography

Periprocedural TEE can visualize pericardial effusions in real-time. Perforation of the appendage would immediately cause local hemopericardium of the transverse sinus and left pulmonic recess (Fig. 33). Multiple standard transesophageal views will disclose an abnormal pericardial fluid collection (Fig. 34, Table 2). Standard transthoracic echocardiography views are also available for collateral information on pericardial effusion.[22]

Watchman Device Deployment

Initial examination should assess for the presence of LAA thrombus, which precludes the Watchman device (Boston Scientific, Natick, MA, USA) deployment, pericardial effusion (moderate or greater an exclusion criteria), and left ventricular ejection fraction (<30% exclusion criteria).

Multiplane sweep views of the LAA at 0, 45, 90, and 135° are performed to determine the maximal measurements of the LAA ostium diameter and width, and length of the primary lobe (Fig. 35).

Depending on the LAA configuration and particular location of the cutting plane relative to the centroid point of the appendage, the short axis of the left coronary artery and the "coumadin ridge," also known as the left upper left pulmonary

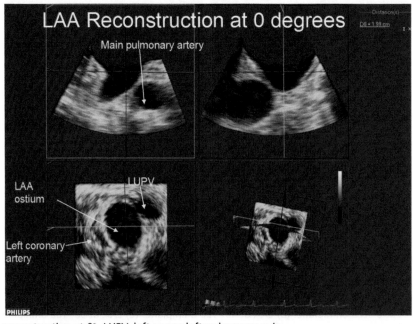

Fig. 37. LAA reconstruction at 0°. LUPV, left upper left pulmonary vein.

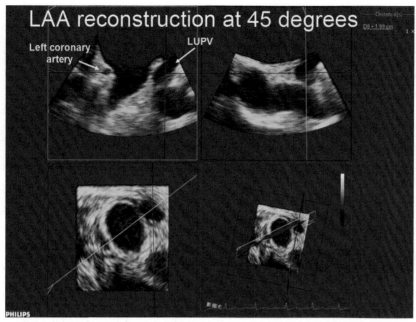

Fig. 38. LAA reconstruction along the 45° omniplane (*green line*) includes both the left coronary artery in short axis and the LUPV.

vein (LUPV) limbus or Marshall ligament, may be visualized (**Fig. 36**). When these structures are identified, the diameter of the LAA should be measured from the left coronary artery to a point approximately 2 cm from the tip of the LUPV (in this example, at 45° and 90° **Figs. 37** and **38**).

Otherwise, the measurement should be obtained from the top of the mitral valve annulus to a point approximately 2 cm from the tip of the LUPV limbus. The approximate LAA length from the ostium line to the apex of the LAA should be measured.

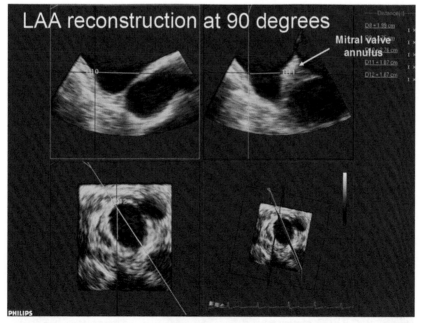

Fig. 39. The LAA ostium diameter measured in the 90° plane (*green line*) can often be the largest diameter depending on shape of the LAA ostium.

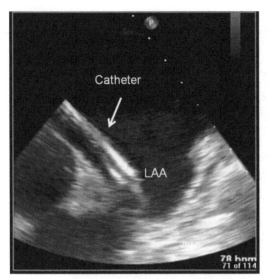

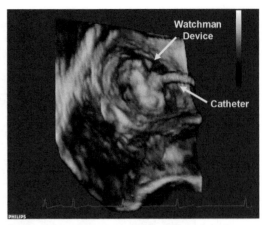

Fig. 42. 3D en-face view of the deployed device.

Fig. 40. The delivery catheter should be advanced into the main LAA lobe under TEE guidance.

In general, a device 20% bigger than the maximum measurement is chosen.

3D TEE is a useful adjunct to 2D TEE imaging, especially in confirming sizing or irregular LAA anatomy. The 3D LAA view from above from the LA is particularly useful as the reference view before cropping and further analysis. The key structures to be recognized are the LAA ostium (the shape of which is usually oval, as seen in

Fig. 36), the LUPV, and the LUPV limbus (or Marshall ligament).

In the 0° (transverse) plane section (green line left lower quadrant), the LUPV is observed in the posterolateral aspect and the left coronary artery in the anteromedial aspect relative to the LAA ostium. This view illustrates why a 0° section through the center of the LAA ostium (corresponding to the 2D image in **Fig. 4**) will not include the LUPV and the left coronary artery (**Fig. 37**). LAA reconstruction along the 45° omniplane (green line in **Fig. 38**) includes both the left coronary artery in short axis and the LUPV. The LAA ostium diameter measured in the 90° plane (green line in

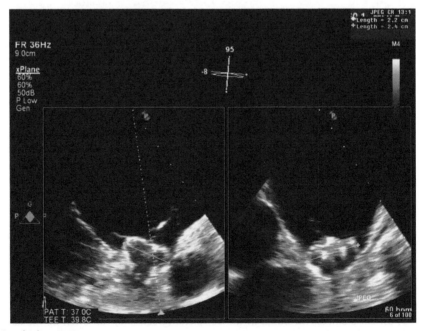

Fig. 41. Device deployment.

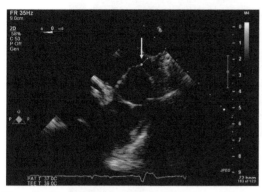

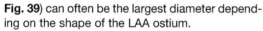

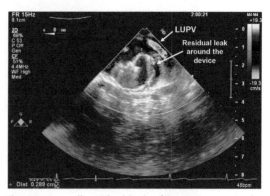

Fig. 43. Significant gap (*arrow*) seen between Watchman device (Boston Scientific) and lateral LAA wall displayed at 0°.

Fig. 44. A small residual leak of 3 mm is seen in the posterosuperior aspect of the device adjacent to the LUPV limbus.

Fig. 39) can often be the largest diameter depending on the shape of the LAA ostium.

The delivery catheter should be advanced into the main LAA lobe under TEE guidance (**Fig. 40**) and swept from 0° to 135° to observe device position from all views/angles.

The Watchman device should be positioned at or distal to the LAA ostium and can protrude only slightly into the LAA. If the device position is too proximal (significant protrusion of device into the LA) or too distal, the device should be fully recaptured, removed, and replaced. All lobes of the LAA

should be covered with the device. Maximum diameter of device "shoulders" at multiple angles should be measured (green lines). Ideal device size after deployment should measure approximately 80% to 90% of its original size (corresponding to a compression of 10%–20%) (**Fig. 41**). Inappropriate compression may require device repositioning or resizing.

3D imaging provides an en-face view of the device deployed in the LAA. This view demonstrates the slight protrusion into the LA and the catheter, which is still attached to the device (**Fig. 42**).

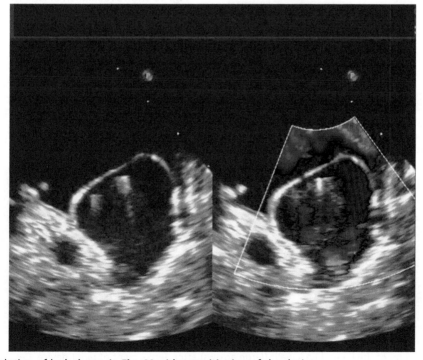

Fig. 45. Resolution of leak shown in **Fig. 44** with repositioning of the device.

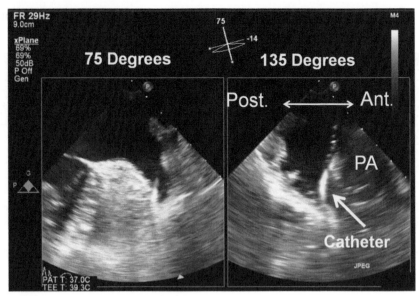

Fig. 46. The anterioposterior view of the LAA is best displayed in the 110°–135° TEE omniplane view. Ant., anterior; PA, pulmonary artery; Post., posterior.

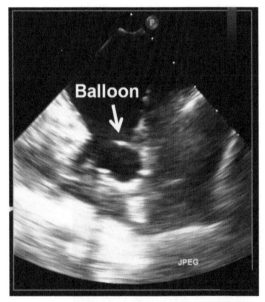

Fig. 47. Once the catheter has been placed in the anterior portion or lobe of the LAA, a balloon is inflated to determine proper positioning of the Lariat snare.

Watchman Improper Positioning

Fig. 43 shows significant gap (arrow) between Watchman device and lateral LAA wall displayed at 0°.

Fig. 44 demonstrates a small residual leak of 3 mm in the posterosuperior aspect of the device adjacent to the LUPV limbus. Significant flow around device edge (>5 mm in diameter) or significant flow into any uncovered secondary lobe is a suboptimal result and may require device repositioning or resizing.

Fig. 45 shows resolution of leak with repositioning of the device.

Lariat Device Implantation

An important role for echocardiography during Lariat device (SentreHeart, Redwood City, CA, USA) LAA ligation is to guide the catheter into the more anteriorly positioned lobe. The anterior-posterior view of the LAA is best displayed in the 110° to 135° TEE omniplane view. In this view,

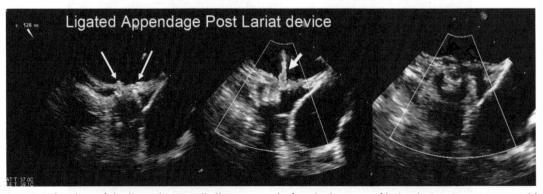

Fig. 48. Left, edges of the ligated LAA walls (*large arrows*) after deployment of lariat device. Center, trace residual low-velocity flow (*short arrow*) from LAA body before tightening of the suture. Right, resolution of residual flow from LAA body after tightening of suture.

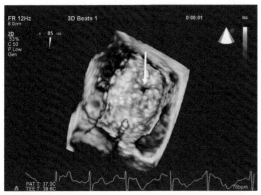

Fig. 49. 3D TEE image of the en-face view of LAA after ligation with Lariat device. Arrow points to central "dimple" representing the residual orifice of the ligated LAA.

the pulmonary artery can often be visualized to the right of the appendage and is a landmark for anterior orientation (**Fig. 46**).

Once the catheter has been placed in the anterior portion or lobe of the LAA, a balloon is inflated to determine proper positioning of the Lariat snare (**Fig. 47**).

Fig. 48 shows edges of the ligated LAA walls (left panel, large arrows) after deployment of the Lariat device; the middle panel shows trace residual low-velocity flow from LAA body before tightening of the suture. Resolution of residual flow from LAA body after tightening of the suture is shown in the right panel. The 3D TEE image shows the en-face view of LAA following ligation with Lariat device. The arrow points to a central "dimple" representing the residual orifice of the ligated LAA (**Fig. 49**).

REFERENCES

1. Al-Saady NM, Obel OA, Camm AJ. Left atrial appendage: structure, function, and role in thromboembolism. Heart 1999;82:547–55.
2. Veinot JP, Harrity PJ, Gentile F, et al. Anatomy of the normal left atrial appendage: a quantitative study of age-related changes in 500 autopsy hearts: implications for echocardiographic examination. Circulation 1997;96:3112–5.
3. Di Biase L, Santangeli P, Anselmino M, et al. Does the left atrial appendage morphology correlate with the risk of stroke in patients with atrial fibrillation? J Am Coll Cardiol 2012;60:531–8.
4. Ho SY, Caea JA, Sanchez-Quina D. Left atrial anatomy revisited. Circ Arrhythm Electrophysiol 2012;5:220–8.
5. Pollick C, Taylor D. Assessment of left atrial appendage function by transesophageal echocardiography.

Implications for the development of thrombus. Circulation 1991;84:223–31.
6. Ho SY, Basso C, Cabrera JA, et al. Anatomy of structures relevant to atrial fibrillation ablation. Chapter 1. In: Natale A, Raviele A, editors. Atrial Fibrillation Ablation, 2011 Update: The State of the Art based on the VeniceChart International Consensus Document. New York: Wiley-Blackwell; 2011. p. 1–19.
7. Su P, McCarthy KP, Ho SY. Occluding the left atrial appendage: anatomical considerations. Heart 2007;94:1166–70.
8. Nucifora G, Faletra FF, Regoli F, et al. Evaluation of the left atrial appendage with real-time 3-dimensional transesophageal echocardiography: implications for catheter-based left atrial appendage closure. Circ Cardiovasc Imaging 2011;4:514–23.
9. Groell R, Schlaffer GJ, Rienmueller R. pericardial sinuses and recesses: findings at electrocardiographically triggered electron-beam CT. Radiology 1999;212:69–73.
10. Agmon Y, Khandheria BK, Gentile F, et al. Echocardiographic assessment of the left atrial appendage. J Am Coll Cardiol 1999;34:1867–77.
11. Willens HJ, Qin JH, Keih K, et al. Diagnosis of a bilobed left atrial appendage and pectinate muscles mimicking thrombi on real-time 3-dimensional transesophageal echocardiography. J Ultrasound Med 2010;29:975–80.
12. Donal E, Yamada H, Leclercq C, et al. The left atrial appendage, a small, blind-ended structure: a review of its echocardiographic evaluation and its clinical role. Chest 2005;128:1853–62.
13. The Stroke Prevention in Atrial Fibrillation Investigators Committee on Echocardiography. Transesophageal echocardiographic correlates of thromboembolism in high-risk patients with nonvalvular atrial fibrillation. Ann Intern Med 1998;128(8):639–47.
14. Antonielli E, Pizzuit A, Palinkas A, et al. Clinical value of left atrial appendage flow for prediction of long-term sinus rhythm maintenance in patients with nonvalvular atrial fibrillation. J Am Coll Cardiol 2002;39:1443–9.
15. Goldman ME, Pearce LA, Hart RG, et al. Pathophysiologic correlates of thromboembolism in nonvalvular atrial fibrillation: I. Reduced flow. J Am Soc Echocardiogr 1999;12:1080–7 Velocity in the Left Atrial Appendage (The Stroke Prevention in Atrial Fibrillation [SPAF-III] Study).
16. Kamalesh M, Copeland TB, Sawada S. Severely reduced left atrial appendage function: a cause of embolic stroke in patients in sinus rhythm? J Am Soc Echocardiogr 1998;11:902–4.
17. Palinka A, Antonielli E, Picano E, et al. Clinical value of left atrial appendage flow velocity for predicting of cardioversion success in patients with non-valvular atrial fibrillation. Eur Heart J 2001;22:2201–8.

18. Ilercil A, Kondapaneni J, Hla A, et al. Influence of age on left atrial appendage function in patients with nonvalvular atrial fibrillation. Clin Cardiol 2001; 24:39–44.

19. Tabata T, Oki T, Fukuda N, et al. Influence of aging on left atrial appendage flow velocity patterns in normal subjects. J Am Soc Echocardiogr 1996;9: 274–80.

20. Faletra FF, Nucifora G, Ho SY. Imaging the atrial septum using real-time three-dimensional transesophageal echocardiography: technical tips, normal anatomy, and its role in transseptal puncture. J Am Soc Echocardiogr 2011;24:593–9.

21. Perk G, Lang RM, Garcia-Fernandez MA, et al. Use of real time three-dimensional transesophageal echocardiography in intracardiac catheter based interventions. J Am Soc Echocardiogr 2009;22: 865–82.

22. Dudzinski DM, Mak G, Hung J. Pericardial disease. Curr Probl Cardiol 2012;37:75–118.

Pericardial Access for LARIAT Left Atrial Appendage Closure

Miguel Valderrábano, MD

KEYWORDS

- Anterior pericardial puncture • LARIAT left atrial appendage procedure • LARIAT LAA

KEY POINTS

- Anterior pericardial puncture requires intimate knowledge of the mediastinal anatomy and careful review of the individual anatomic characteristics of each patient.
- Familiarity with the procedure's anatomic foundations and with the basic principles of each procedural step are critical, but once this is achieved, the procedure is safe and in most cases, preferable to a standard inferior puncture.
- An uncomplicated and properly placed pericardial puncture is the basis of a successful LARIAT procedure.
- Operators must master the intricacies of the anterior pericardial puncture before embarking on LARIAT left atrial appendage ligation.

INTRODUCTION: NATURE OF THE PROBLEM

Since its original description in 1996 by Sosa and colleagues,[1] percutaneous access to the pericardial sac for therapeutic purposes has gradually become a commonplace procedure in the electrophysiology laboratory. Initially devised for the treatment of ventricular tachycardias in the setting of Chagas disease,[2,3] its use for the treatment of ischemic ventricular tachycardia[4] expanded the clinical spectrum of patients that could benefit from mapping and ablating arrhythmia substrates in the epicardial aspect of the heart to a broad range of conditions, including accessory pathways,[5,6] atrial tachycardias,[5] and ventricular tachycardias in the setting of right ventricular dysplasia.[7–9] Over the years, an anterior puncture variation[10] has evolved that is particularly suited for the LARIAT suture delivery device (SentreHEART, Inc, Redwood City, CA, USA) procedure.

The LARIAT sutured-based procedure capitalizes on this large collective[8] experience for the purpose of epicardial ligation of the left atrial appendage (LAA). Important anatomic considerations apply when routine pericardial access is adapted to instrumentation of the LAA.

ANATOMIC CONSIDERATIONS: LOCATION OF THE LAA WITHIN THE PERICARDIAL SAC AND RELEVANCE OF THE PUNCTURE SITE

The outer layer of the pericardial sac is the parietal pericardium, which is continuous with the visceral pericardium via reflections in the great vessels. The pericardial sac normally contains sufficient pericardial fluid circumferentially so as to allow entrance in the pericardial space without puncturing the heart at any location of the sac. When the goal of entering the pericardial space is to reach the LAA, the point of entrance is critical. Depending on where the pericardial sac is punctured, delivering a catheter or a wire to the area of the LAA may be easy or impossible, due to the presence of anatomic structures that may be interposed between the puncture site and the LAA. Thus, it is critical to understand the location of the LAA within the pericardial sac. **Fig. 1** shows

The author has nothing to disclose.
Division of Cardiac Electrophysiology, Department of Cardiology, Methodist DeBakey Heart and Vascular Center, Houston Methodist Hospital, Baylor College of Medicine, Weill College of Medicine, Cornell University, 6550 Fannin Street, Suite 1901, Houston, TX 77030, USA
E-mail address: MValderrabano@houstonmethodist.org

Intervent Cardiol Clin 3 (2014) 281–289
http://dx.doi.org/10.1016/j.iccl.2013.12.003
2211-7458/14/$ – see front matter © 2014 Elsevier Inc. All rights reserved.

interventional.theclinics.com

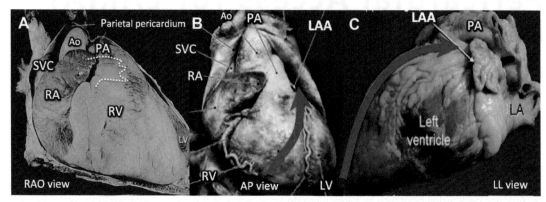

Fig. 1. General anatomy of the pericardial sac as related to the LAA. (*A*) Open pericardial sac with the heart in situ viewed at an angle comparable to a fluoroscopic right anterior oblique (RAO) projection. The right ventricle (RV) dominates the visualized portion of the heart, and the LAA location is marked by the white dotted line. (*B*) In an anteroposterior (AP) view, only the tip of the LAA can be visualized lateral to the pulmonary artery (PA). (*C*) In a left lateral (LL) view, the LAA is all the way posterior, inferior, and lateral to the pulmonary artery. The red arrow illustrates the course of the pericardial catheterization required to reach the LAA from an anterior puncture. Ao, aorta; LA, left atrium; LV, left ventricle; RA, right atrium; SVC, superior vena cava.

these anatomic relationships in the human heart inside the pericardial sac viewed in different angles comparable to those of conventional fluoroscopic views. In a right anterior oblique view (see **Fig. 1**, left panel) the LAA is not visible behind the pulmonary artery (outlined by the dotted line). In an anteroposterior view, only the LAA tip is visible to the left of the pulmonary artery. A left lateral view illustrates how posterior the LAA body is, posterior and lateral to the pulmonary artery.

From these images, the ideal trajectory of a catheter aiming to reach the LAA is clear, illustrated by the red arrows. A straight pathway is important to maximize transmission of catheter manipulation maneuvers (ie, deflection, torque, and so forth) onto the catheter tip. Thus, to achieve this trajectory, the most favorable puncture site is the anterior wall of the pericardial sac, aiming to enter the pericardial space in front of the right ventricle, and directing the needle toward the LAA in the cardiac silhouette. **Fig. 2** shows an example. In the frontal plane, the goal is to enter the pericardium where it is most anterior (see later in this article) and direct the needle toward 1 in the clock phase, so that when the sheath is advanced, it will be lateral to the pulmonary artery. If the puncture aims too medial, the pulmonary artery will obstruct the trajectory toward the LAA. If the puncture is too lateral, the sheath will tend to go low toward the lateral wall of the left ventricle.

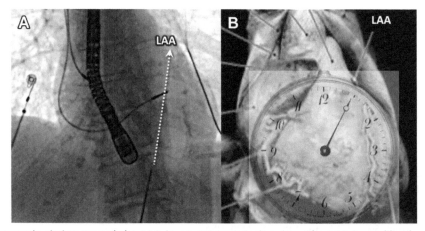

Fig. 2. Fluoroscopic aiming toward the LAA in an anteroposterior view. The LAA is readily identified in the cardiac silhouette as the prominence below the pulmonary artery shadow (*A*). To reach it, the puncture must be oriented toward the 1 o'clock phase (*B*).

PREPROCEDURAL PLANNING

There are significant anatomic variations that need to be assessed before the procedure. Certain characteristics of the LAA anatomy on cardiac computerized tomography (CT) scan may completely preclude delivery of the LARIAT snare and patients with such anatomies will be excluded. But even for patients with suitable anatomies, a thorough review of the cardiac CT is warranted to understand the individual anatomic relationships. **Figs. 3** and **4** show examples of the insights gained by CT, which include the tightness of the substernal space anterior to the right ventricle (see **Fig. 3**A), the width of the LAA and possible superior course (see **Fig. 3**B), the size of the pulmonary artery and its overlap with the LAA (see **Fig. 3**C), and the extent of costo-chondral hypertrophy and length of the xyphoid process (see **Fig. 3**D). The anatomic variations of the xyphoid process are of specific relevance to the pericardial puncture access site. **Fig. 4** shows some of these. The triangle form between the lower ribs on both sides and the sternum is occupied by the xyphoid process. This can be small (see **Fig. 4**A), leaving sufficient space to visualize the pericardial sac underneath, or large (see **Fig. 4**B), completely obliterating the triangle, and forcing consideration

of a lower puncture. In obese patients, the prominent abdomen can cause upward curvature of the xyphoid process (see **Fig. 4**C), and may make it impossible to keep a shallow angle of the needle. In these cases, a lower puncture may be of help (see later in this article).

THE ANTERIOR PERICARDIAL PUNCTURE

For the desired sheath trajectory, it is critical to enter the pericardium in its most anterior aspect, immediately under the sternum. A left lateral fluoroscopic view is critical to guide the needle positioning. The left lateral view provides important information as to the anatomic relationship between the pericardial sac and the retrosternal space. This view will be used to advance the needle from the subxyphoid skin puncture immediately under the sternum.

It is important to create a shallow needle angulation after the needle is underneath the xyphoid process, so that it advances in the retrosternal space in the mediastinum, anterior to the pericardial sac and posterior to the sternum. In obese patients with prominent abdomens, it can be challenging to keep a shallow needle angle. Contrast is injected to verify the position of the needle as it is advanced. The lateral view is used to enter this

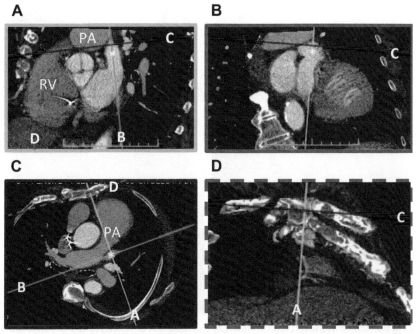

Fig. 3. Anatomic relationships of the sternum, pericardial sac, and LAA demonstrated by CT. (*A*) Sagittal slice at the level of the LAA (*asterisk*) posteriorly and the xyphoid process anteriorly. A tight contact between the sternum (*left*) and the right ventricle (RV) can be appreciated. (*B*) Coronal slice at the level of the LAA (*asterisk*). (*C*) Axial slice at the level of the LAA (*asterisk*), showing its intimate connection to the pulmonary artery (PA). (*D*) Coronal slice at the level of the xyphoid process. Colored lines indicate respective planes of each slice.

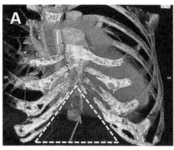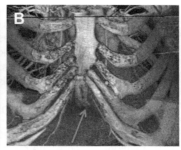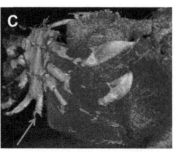

Fig. 4. Anatomic variations of the xyphoid process. It occupies the triangle between the lower ribs (*white dotted triangle*). (*A*) A small, atrophied xyphoid process leaves an empty triangle with the pericardial sac directly underneath. (*B*) A large xyphoid process obliterates the triangle, which would require a lower puncture. (*C*) Large, hypertrophied, and curved xyphoid process in an obese patient. *Arrow* shows the location where the needle would be advanced.

space, maintaining a shallow angle to avoid direct right ventricular puncture. This view is also critical to avoid puncturing the pericardial sac in the subdiaphragmatic (inferior) region. A subdiaphragmatic puncture will lead the wire and lead toward the inferolateral left ventricle, in an angulation most unfavorable to reach the LAA. **Fig. 5** shows an example. In this view, the apex

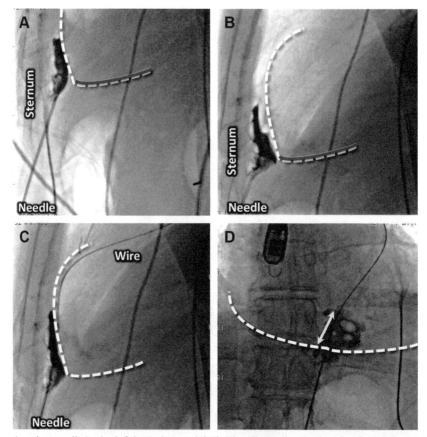

Fig. 5. Advancing the needle in the left lateral view. (*A*) The needle is advanced under the sternum with a shallow angle to avoid the diaphragmatic aspect of the pericardial sac (*red line*). Except in very obese patients, the pericardial sac is usually identifiable (*white dotted line*). Contrast is injected. (*B*) The needle is advanced toward the heart, creating tenting in the pocket of contrast. (*C*) The wire is advanced and followed into the pericardial sac. (*D*) In the anteroposterior view, the needle and contrast are well past the cardiac silhouette (*yellow arrow*), and it is impossible to ascertain the depth of the needle or to diagnose a possible right ventricular perforation.

of the heart is clearly visible, marking an acute angle formed by the diaphragmatic aspect of the pericardial sac (marked as a red line) and its anterior aspect. The needle must be inserted in the retrosternal space between the anterior aspect of the pericardial sac and the sternum. A puncture in the diaphragmatic aspect of the pericardial sac would commit the wire and sheath to an inferolateral course that would make it impossible to reach the LAA.

The relevance of the lateral view is obvious when compared with an anteroposterior view (see **Fig. 5**D), where contrast will be seen in front of the cardiac silhouette. In the lateral view, contrast injection creates a dense pocket of contrast in front of the pericardial sac. It is important to verify that the pocket of contrast has gentle cardiac motions transmitted from the adjacent pericardial sac. If cardiac motion is absent, the needle may be too shallow in the retrosternal space. In the anteroposterior view, this pocket of contrast lies in front of the cardiac silhouette, in an image that shows the needle past the silhouette that could be indistinguishable from a perforation.

Once a pocket of contrast is created between the sternum and the anterior aspect of the pericardial sac, the needle will be used to puncture it. The obvious difficulty is to puncture only the sac and not the underlying right ventricle. Several steps can be taken to perform this successfully. It is helpful to keep the bevel of the needle pointing toward the sternum so that the blunt side of the needle faces the pericardial sac (**Fig. 6**). Once the needle tip is at the desired location, its angulation

will be made steeper to create a tent in the pocket of contrast toward the pericardial sac. Firmly holding the needle in a fixed position while tenting the sac for a few respiratory cycles may be sufficient to puncture the sac, as the very respiratory motion may help perforate the tented parietal pericardium. Alternatively, respirations may be held and the needle then advanced against only the cardiac motion. Additional maneuvers that can help include rotating the needle, introducing a stylet, or steepening the needle angulation. Advancing the needle in the cephalad direction may help find another spot in which to puncture. Obviously, these maneuvers must be performed under careful fluoroscopic visualization at the left lateral view.

On successful puncturing, contrast layering in front of the right ventricle will be evident. **Fig. 7** shows an example. Once again, a lateral fluoroscopic angle is critical to appreciate the layering. In other angles, contrast diffuses indistinctly. Once contrast layering is identified, the wire will be advanced. The course of the wire as it advances in the chest must be carefully inspected to verify that it stays within the limits of the cardiac silhouette. Wire advancement outside the cardiac silhouette indicates either pleural or right ventricular puncture (see later in this article).

POTENTIAL DIFFICULTIES AND COMPLICATIONS
Adhesions

Prior pericardial inflammation, clinical or subclinical, radiation to the chest, or chronic renal failure

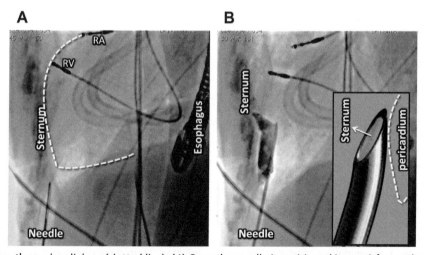

Fig. 6. Tenting the pericardial sac (*dotted line*). (*A*) Once the needle is positioned in a satisfactory location in the retrosternal space, its angle is steepened to create tenting. The cardiac motion will be felt by the hand holding the needle. (*B*) Safest needle orientation to avoid right ventricular perforation. The bevel is oriented anteriorly toward the sternum (*inset*). RA, right atrium; RV, right ventricle.

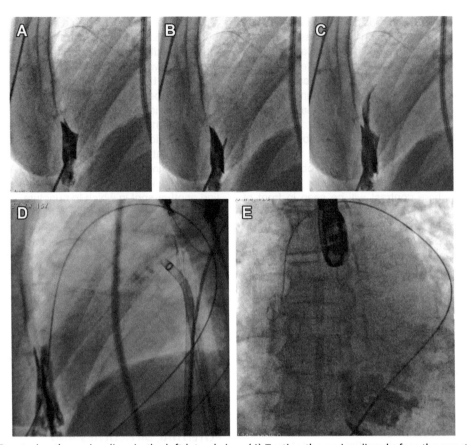

Fig. 7. Puncturing the pericardium in the left lateral view. (*A*) Tenting the pericardium before the puncture. (*B*) Immediately after puncture, the tenting is released and needle is beyond the pocket of contrast. Note the oblique upward angle of needle advancement. (*C*) Contrast is injected and layering around the right ventricular surface is seen. (*D*) The wire is advanced and it follows the cardiac silhouette. (*E*) In the anteroposterior view, the wire remains in the pericardial sac within the cardiac silhouette.

may be associated with a scarring process in the pericardial space leading to adhesions of the visceral and parietal pericardium. Pericardial adhesions can be noticed as contrast is injected after pericardial puncture. Instead of contrast layering, the fluoroscopic image will show a well-delimited pocket within the pericardial sac without diffusing across the pericardial space. **Fig. 8** shows an example. This is not an uncommon problem for operators experienced in electrophysiological applications of the pericardial puncture. It is possible to release the adhesions, to a certain extent, by introducing a wire or even an ablation catheter to expand the pocket and reach the LAA. **Fig. 8** shows how releasing the adhesions can be performed to enable advancing the epicardial wire all the way to the LAA and achieve connection of the epicardial and endocardial wires. However, this usually is a meaningless partial success, because pericardial adhesions are uniformly and consistently associated with adhesions around the LAA itself that will make it impossible to

advance the LARIAT snare (see **Fig. 8**F) and ultimately lead to procedure failure. Thus, it is recommended that in the presence of adhesions, the procedure be abandoned promptly rather than subjecting the patient to futile, eventually unsuccessful, attempts.

Entry That Is Too Medial or Too Lateral

When access to the pericardial sac is too medial, the pulmonary artery will obstruct passage of the LARIAT snare toward the LAA. If this is the case, a second puncture may be required. Most commonly, the decision to require a second puncture is made after an initial puncture has been made and has failed to allow successful LARIAT delivery and after a trans-septal puncture has been performed and anticoagulation has been initiated. Thus, a second puncture most commonly would be performed under anticoagulation. Although this is not an absolute contraindication, pericardial access under anticoagulation does

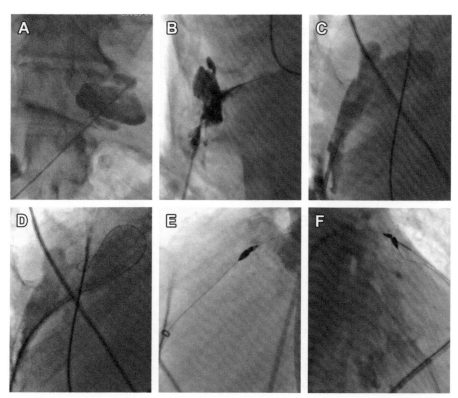

Fig. 8. Pericardial adhesions. (*A, B*) Sharply delimited pockets of contrast in the anteroposterior or lateral view may indicate the presence of adhesions. (*C*) Contrast injection in the pericardium confirms the presence of loculated adhesions as it remains in an isolated pocket. (*D*) The adhesions may be released with a wire or an ablation catheter, even allowing advancement of the magnetic-tip wire toward the LAA, as seen in *E*. However, adhesions around the LAA precluded advancement of the LARIAT, as seen in *F*, and eventually led to procedure failure.

increase the risk of bleeding in the event of a right ventricular perforation (see later in this article).

Pleural Puncture

In certain patients, the left lung pleural reflections may reach the anterior mediastinum. If this is the case, typically the pleural reflections lie anterior to the pericardial sac, between it and the sternum. It is possible to puncture the pleural space. **Fig. 9** shows an example. Most commonly, the lung parenchyma is not involved, and there would be no adverse consequences of pericardial entry. Careful monitoring for the possible development of pneumothorax is nevertheless advisable. Pleural puncture may be anticipated if after substernal contrast injection the needle tents but there are no cardiac motions transmitted onto the pocket of contrast.

Right Ventricular Perforation

Given the close anatomic relationships, right ventricular perforation is an inherent risk of the

pericardial puncture. If properly recognized, it is not necessarily of adverse consequences. Clues to a right ventricular perforation include (1) rapid dissipation of contrast from the needle tip as it is pumped toward the pulmonary artery, (2) pulsatile blood return from the needle, (3) wire advancement toward the pulmonary artery past the cardiac silhouette, or (4) endovascular wire inside the pulmonary artery on transesophageal echocardiography. In the event of a right ventricular perforation, the needle will be retracted gently and redirected in a more shallow angle while probing with the wire. Once the wire is seen to advance into the pericardial space, it is advisable to drain any pericardial blood and observe under echocardiography for the development of pericardial effusion for a few minutes before proceeding. In the absence of anticoagulation, most right ventricular perforations are of no consequence and would seal spontaneously, but careful monitoring is required before proceeding with the rest of the procedure. Failure to recognize a right ventricular perforation can be catastrophic if serial dilatations

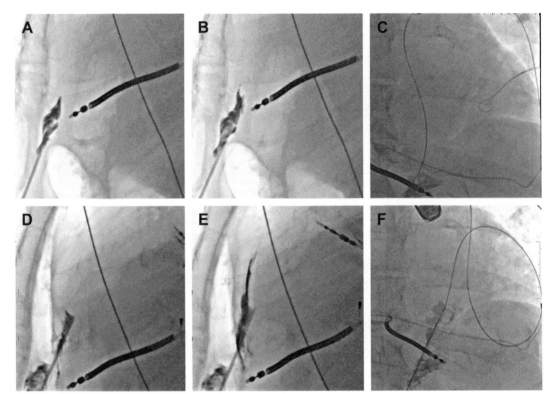

Fig. 9. Pleural puncture. In patients with prominent medial pleural reflections, a shallow puncture (*A*) under the sternum may lead to layering of contrast (*B*), leading to the belief that pericardial access has been achieved. However, the wire will advance beyond the cardiac silhouette into the pleural space (*C*). A clue to pleural puncture is the lack of cardiac motion during the initial tenting and needle advancement. In the same case, a steeper needle angle reached the pericardial sac (*D*) and punctured the pericardium successfully (*E*), as shown by the wire's final position within the pericardial sac (*F*).

are performed, leading to a large sheath insertion into the right ventricular cavity. If that happens, prompt surgical consultation should be obtained *before* pulling the sheath out of the right ventricle.

Additional Complications

As with any pericardial puncture and instrumentation of the pericardial space, additional complications may occur. Overall complication rates range between 5% and 8%.[11,12] These include pericarditis (which can be chronic or recurrent), hemopericardium, hemoperitoneum, adbomino-pericardial fistula,[13] liver/spleen laceration, gut laceration, coronary vein/artery laceration, and subdiaphragmatic vessel injury. Damage to abdominal contents can be prevented by the anterior approach and the use of the lateral fluoroscopic view.[14] Careful fluoroscopic monitoring and a scrupulous technique may help prevent some of these complications, which are known to occur early in the operator's experience.[13] Additionally, the use of an ultrathin needle for the initial puncture (21G) may help prevent myocardial punctures.

SUMMARY

Anterior pericardial puncture requires intimate knowledge of the mediastinal anatomy and careful review of the individual anatomic characteristics of each patient. Familiarity with the procedure's anatomic foundations and with the basic principles of each procedural step are critical, but once this is achieved, the procedure is safe and, in most cases, preferable to a standard inferior puncture. An uncomplicated and properly placed pericardial puncture is the basis of a successful LARIAT procedure. Operators must master the intricacies of the anterior pericardial puncture before embarking on LARIAT LAA ligation.

REFERENCES

1. Sosa E, Scanavacca M, d'Avila A, et al. A new technique to perform epicardial mapping in the electrophysiology laboratory. J Cardiovasc Electrophysiol 1996;7:531–6.

2. Sosa E, Scanavacca M, D'Avila A, et al. Endocardial and epicardial ablation guided by nonsurgical

transthoracic epicardial mapping to treat recurrent ventricular tachycardia. J Cardiovasc Electrophysiol 1998;9:229–39.

3. Scanavacca M, Sosa E, D'Avila A, et al. Radiofrequency catheter ablation in patients with atrial fibrillation. Arq Bras Cardiol 1999;72:693–708.

4. Sosa E, Scanavacca M, d'Avila A, et al. Nonsurgical transthoracic epicardial catheter ablation to treat recurrent ventricular tachycardia occurring late after myocardial infarction. J Am Coll Cardiol 2000;35: 1442–9.

5. Schweikert RA, Saliba WI, Tomassoni G, et al. Percutaneous pericardial instrumentation for endo-epicardial mapping of previously failed ablations. Circulation 2003;108:1329–35.

6. Valderrabano M, Cesario DA, Ji S, et al. Percutaneous epicardial mapping during ablation of difficult accessory pathways as an alternative to cardiac surgery. Heart Rhythm 2004;1:311–6.

7. Bai R, Di Biase L, Shivkumar K, et al. Ablation of ventricular arrhythmias in arrhythmogenic right ventricular dysplasia/cardiomyopathy: arrhythmia-free survival after endo-epicardial substrate based mapping and ablation. Circ Arrhythm Electrophysiol 2011;4:478–85.

8. Della Bella P, Brugada J, Zeppenfeld K, et al. Epicardial ablation for ventricular tachycardia: a European multicenter study. Circ Arrhythm Electrophysiol 2011;4:653–9.

9. Haqqani HM, Tschabrunn CM, Betensky BP, et al. Layered activation of epicardial scar in arrhythmogenic right ventricular dysplasia: possible substrate for confined epicardial circuits. Circ Arrhythm Electrophysiol 2012;5:796–803.

10. Jais P, Maury P, Khairy P, et al. Elimination of local abnormal ventricular activities: a new end point for substrate modification in patients with scar-related ventricular tachycardia. Circulation 2012; 125:2184–96.

11. Sacher F, Roberts-Thomson K, Maury P, et al. Epicardial ventricular tachycardia ablation: a multicenter safety study. J Am Coll Cardiol 2010;55: 2366–72.

12. Tung R, Michowitz Y, Yu R, et al. Epicardial ablation of ventricular tachycardia: an institutional experience of safety and efficacy. Heart Rhythm 2013;10: 490–8.

13. Killu AM, Friedman PA, Mulpuru SK, et al. Atypical complications encountered with epicardial electrophysiological procedures. Heart Rhythm 2013;10: 1613–21.

14. Weerasooriya R, Jais P, Sacher F, et al. Utility of the lateral fluoroscopic view for subxiphoid pericardial access. Circ Arrhythm Electrophysiol 2009;2:e15–7.

Clinical Results with Percutaneous Left Atrial Appendage Occlusion

Zoltan G. Turi, MD

KEYWORDS

• Atrial fibrillation • Left atrial appendage • Anticoagulation • Cardiac catheterization

KEY POINTS

- Closure of the left atrial appendage (LAA) is associated with significant reduction in embolic events; this is likely to be device independent.
- There is an initial hazard associated with closure methodologies; once successful closure is achieved the results appear to be superior to those of anticoagulation.
- The evidence base is largely limited to the safety and efficacy of LAA occlusion in patients who are candidates for anticoagulation as well.
- The risk to benefit ratio of competing closure technologies has not been determined.
- In patients with high embolic risk and high risk of anticoagulation, LAA occlusion plus antiplatelet therapy seems to have an acceptable therapeutic and safety profile.

INTRODUCTION
Background

Although left atrial appendage (LAA) occlusion has been performed in the surgical arena for more than a half century, there is virtually no higher-level evidence base from that vast operative experience. Clinical outcomes data are largely confined to the literature of the last half decade and derive almost exclusively from the percutaneous approach. Thus, it was assumed but not proved that LAA occlusion decreases the risk of thromboembolism in atrial fibrillation, and that surgical ligation, clipping, or amputation have favorable therapeutic benefits. The surgical literature incorporates just 1 prematurely abandoned randomized trial without significant outcomes data.[1] The emergence of percutaneous LAA occlusion, with an accompanying high-level evidence base, is revolutionizing our understanding of the role of the LAA in thromboembolic disease and clarifying the influence of excluding the LAA on outcomes.

Despite the absence of randomized trials in the surgical literature, the surgical experience has yielded important insights into the modern clinical trials. Oversewing, or ligating, the LAA dates to at least 1949, when Bailey and colleagues,[2] who pioneered the modern era of heart surgery, noted thrombus in the LAA with subsequent fatal cerebral embolization after mitral commissurotomy. This was the fourth case in their series, after which for a time they routinely if empirically performed left atrial ligation. There was controversy regarding the usefulness of LAA ligation, and an alternative approach during heart surgery, which involved manipulation of the appendage and temporary occlusion of the left common carotid and innominate arteries, was considered.[3] Over the subsequent several decades, LAA exclusion was inconsistently applied to a variety of procedures in which patients had valve surgery, in particular those with atrial fibrillation. The technique was primary suture ligation, with rows of sutures placed from the intra-atrial surface, although stapling and

Disclosure: Z.G. Turi has received research grant support from Boston Scientific (formerly Atritech, Plymouth, MN) and St Jude Medical (St Paul, MN), and has consulted for AtriCure (West Chester, OH).
Department of Medicine, Rutgers Robert Wood Johnson Medical School, One Robert Wood Johnson Place, MEB 582A New Brunswick, NJ 08903, USA
E-mail address: zoltan.turi@rutgers.edu

interventional.theclinics.com

external loop strangulation were also performed. Amputation has been a less common method although it has increased with the use of automatic clipping and excision devices.[4]

Awareness that there was frequently residual flow into the LAA also stems from the surgical experience, albeit belatedly; the observation that suture ligation in particular was frequently incomplete is relatively recent. Katz and colleagues[5] studied patients undergoing mitral valve repair or replacement and found significant residual flow across suture ligated LAAs in more than a third of patients. This finding appeared to be independent of the size of the left atrium or the size of the LAA. The incidence of incomplete closure was the same in the perioperative setting as during subsequent follow-up, suggesting incomplete closure at the time of surgery rather than subsequent dehiscence. A different ligation technique, use of a purse string from within the left atrium, is also associated with incomplete ligation.[6] The importance of incomplete closure, which is discussed subsequently, remains controversial, but in the surgical series by Katz and colleagues, spontaneous echo contrast in the LAA correlated strongly with incomplete ligation. Besides incomplete suture ligation with residual flow, the presence of a residual stump after stapling was documented in a high percentage of patients in the randomized but prematurely discontinued Left Atrial Appendage Occlusion Study[1] (55% and 28%, respectively), presaging a finding that has been important in the percutaneous LAA occlusion literature. Incomplete occlusion of the LAA by surgery, as high as 60% in 1 series, was associated with a 41% rate of LAA thrombus,[7] also presaging an important concern in the percutaneous LAA closure environment.

Overall Observations Regarding the LAA Closure Literature

Despite widespread use of LAA closure, both in cardiac surgery as well as more recently with a variety of percutaneous technologies, this evidence base is incomplete. Only the PROTECT AF (WATCHMAN Left Atrial Appendage System for Embolic Protection in Patients with Atrial Fibrillation) study[8] and PREVAIL (Prospective Randomized Evaluation of the WATCHMAN LAA Closure Device in Patients with Atrial Fibrillation Versus Long-Term Warfarin Therapy) trials[9] were randomized, and the slew of observational studies and registries, with a few exceptions,[10–12] lacked the fundamentals requisite for a higher-level evidence base: multicenter studies with oversight and detailed central data monitoring, core laboratory analyzed data, clinical events committees, and data safety monitoring boards.

The registries, and to a large degree the randomized trials, have depended on historical controls and have suffered from failure of the predicted primary end point event rates to match the observed rates: the CHADS$_2$ score based predictions validated on National Registry of Atrial Fibrillation data[13] have generally been dramatically higher than the observed rates for the controls in the 2 randomized trials. Thus, claims from the observation trials that are entirely based on historical controls have been exaggerated, and the control group in the randomized trials has confounded the statistical analyses. Overall, much of what can definitively be said about LAA closure in general, both device and non–device related, comes from PROTECT AF and PREVAIL.

Percutaneous Approach: Nonrandomized Trial Findings

The concept of percutaneous endocardial LAA occlusion is generally credited to Lesh and van der Burg, whose patent for the PLAATO (Percutaneous Left Atrial Appendage Transcatheter Occlusion) device (ev3 Inc, Plymouth, MN, USA) was granted in 2000. Initial testing in the animal model[14] showed effective LAA occlusion in 25 dogs and endothelialization over a 1-month to 3-month time frame. The time frame for endothelialization in humans seems variable, although a serendipitous event, death from a ruptured abdominal aortic aneurysm with subsequent autopsy examination, yielded confirmation of complete endothelialization of the WATCHMAN device at the time of autopsy, which was 9 months after device placement.[15]

The early trials of LAA occlusion (**Table 1**) were relatively small registries, mostly incorporating patients who were believed to be poor candidates for anticoagulation (except for the WATCHMAN pilot study), and typically included patients with a relatively low CHADS$_2$ score. Before the availability of dedicated LAA occluders, several ad hoc attempts to place devices with other intended uses in the LAA were performed. One published series, by Meier and colleagues,[16] used Amplatzer septal occluders. These investigators reported 1 device embolization, but anecdotal reports of migration from unpublished series strongly suggest that a variety of devices, including atrial and ventricular septal occluders, have a generally unacceptable migration risk. The dedicated LAA devices studied, PLAATO,[17] WATCHMAN (Boston Scientific, Natick, MA, USA),[15] and Amplatzer Cardiac Plug (ACP [St. Jude Medical, Minneapolis, MN, USA]),[18] had variably successful placement (88%–97%) but all

Table 1
Percutaneous LAA occlusion: nonrandomized studies

Reference	Device	Mean Follow-Up	Number of Patients	CHADS$_2$ Score	Successful Placement (%)*	Periprocedural Stroke (%)	Observed Stroke Rate/y	Predicted Stroke Rate/y	Hemopericardium (%)	Embolization (%)
Sievert et al,[19] 2002	PLAATO	1 mo	15		93.8				6.7	0
Ostermayer et al,[17] 2005	PLAATO	9.8 mo	111		95.6	0	2.2	6.3	2.7	0
Sick et al,[15] 2007	WATCHMAN	24 ± 11 mo	75	1.8 ± 1.1	88	0	0	4	2.7	2.7
Park et al,[18] 2011	ACP	0	143		92.3	2.1	N/A	N/A	3.5	2.1
Urena et al,[23] 2013	ACP	20 ± 5 mo	52		98.1	0	1.9		1.9	1.9
Bartus et al,[24] 2013	LARIAT	12 mo	92	1.9 ± 1.0	92.4	0	1.1		3.3	N/A
Follow-up studies										
Park et al,[20] 2009	PLAATO	24 mo	73	2.5 ± 1.4	97.2	0	0	5	0	1.4
Bayard et al,[21] 2010	PLAATO	9.6 ± 6.9 mo	180	3.1 ± 0.8	90	0	2.3	6.6	3.3	0.6
Block et al,[10] 2009	PLAATO	3.75 y	64	2.6	93.9	0	3.8	6.6	1.5	0
Sick et al,[22] 2009	WATCHMAN	58 ± 17 mo	75	1.8 ± 1.1	88	0	0.6	4	2.7	2.7

* Successful placement is based on number of separate catheter laboratory procedures.
Hemopericardium is defined as pericardial effusion undergoing percutaneous or surgical drainage.
Abbreviations: ACP, Amplatzer cardiac plug; N/A, not available or not applicable; PLAATO, percutaneous left atrial appendage transcatheter occluder.

showed dramatic reduction of stroke incidence when compared with historical controls based on predicted event rates associated with CHADS$_2$ scores.[13] All featured a significant complication rate, in particular hemopericardium.

PLAATO

The first series was a small feasibility study of 15 patients reported by Sievert and colleagues[19] in 2002. Although the implantations were all successful (1 patient required 2 separate procedures), there was 1 hemopericardium, and a subsequent 16 patients reported in addendum also had an additional case of hemopericardium, presaging a relatively common and concerning problem associated with LAA occlusion. No randomized trials of the PLAATO device were performed, but there were several subsequent registry reports, most notably by Ostermayer and colleagues,[17] describing 111 patients with attempted implantation. This device was used in patients with relative or absolute contraindications to anticoagulation, and they were treated with antiplatelet therapy only. Again, there were a significant number of patients with hemopericardium, and a dramatic reduction in reported versus predicted stroke risk. Because the PLAATO device was withdrawn, and hence there was no support for follow-up studies, little additional information is available, but limited follow-up was published on both the European[20,21] and North American[10] experience. The larger 180-patient PLAATO study[21] had a 90% success rate, 2 periprocedure deaths, 6 tamponades, and 1 embolization. Successful occlusion was noted in 90%, and the stroke rate was 2.3% per year compared with an expected 6.6%. In the 64-patient North American PLAATO trial,[10] with a mean 3.75-year follow-up, there was a 93.9% success rate, the observed stroke rate was 3.8% versus 6.6% predicted, and there was 1 hemopericardium. Device leak on follow-up transesophageal echocardiography was none to mild in all patients. A 73-patient PLAATO series by Park and colleagues[20] reported a 97.2% success rate. There was 1 device embolization, with the device obstructing the outflow track, resulting in death. There was a common theme in all these studies: substantial reduction in stroke rates from those predicted, and favorable outcomes in patients who had successful device placement. These studies were similarly flawed, and represent at best a modest evidence base for LAA occlusion.

WATCHMAN

The pilot study of the WATCHMAN device by Sick and colleagues[15] had initial 2-year follow-up, again featured significant tamponade risk, and, in addition, had several events common to prototype technologies: there was failure caused by cable breaking and embolization caused by lack of retaining hooks on the device, neither of which occurred after a second-generation WATCHMAN was introduced. The device was placed successfully in 88%; there were 2 tamponades, 3 pericardial effusions, 1 air embolization requiring cardiopulmonary resuscitation, 1 delivery wire fracture, 2 device embolizations, and 4 patients had a thrombus layer at 6 months that resolved with anticoagulation; these observations led to modification of the device as well as the postprocedure use of routine clopidogrel after warfarin discontinuation at 45 days to 6 months. There were 2 transient ischemic attacks: one in a patient who had thrombus noted on the device. Subsequent 58 ± 17 months follow-up revealed a 0.6% annual stroke risk compared with a predicted 4% stroke rate per year.[22] Peridevice flow through a channel less than 3 mm was not considered an adverse outcome, and data on residual leakage are not available. This study, in contrast to most of the other nonrandomized series, featured central core laboratory data assessment, and systematic transesophageal echocardiography, with follow-up for 5 years.

ACP

The evidence base on the ACP device, despite widespread availability for several years outside the United States, remains among the most limited of the LAA technologies. The first significant size series was a retrospective study by Park and colleagues[18] in 2011, which included 143 patients at high risk for anticoagulation, and had only 24 hours of follow-up. Success rate was 92.3%. This series included 2 embolizations, 3 procedure-related strokes, 4 pericardial effusions, and 5 tamponades. Somewhat more evidence base is provided by Urena and colleagues,[23] who assessed 52 patients at 7 Canadian centers with a mean 20 ± 5 months follow-up and reported a 1.9% stroke rate (predicted was 8.6%). It featured 1 embolization, 1 tamponade, and 2 major bleeds in the periprocedure period. Residual peridevice leak was noted in 16% of the patients who had 6 months follow-up; 5 of the 6 patients had new onset of leakage after the initial periprocedure echo.

LARIAT

The LARIAT device is a clever technology, which was approved before the availability of any clinical data; the approval was generic for surgical tissue approximation and not specific for LAA closure. The PLACE II trial[24] describes 92 patients in whom the procedure was attempted; successful placement occurred in 85 (92%). The success rate is similar to a smaller, 27-patient series.[25] There were 3 pericardial effusions in PLACE II that were drained, 3 residual leaks periprocedure, and 4 leaks at 3 months. There were no ischemic strokes at 1-year follow-up. Some concerns regarding PLACE II have been described[26]: it was a single-site study of a low-risk group; less than 5% had a $CHADS_2$ score greater than 3, and nearly half had a $CHADS_2$ score of 1; an unexplained observation relates to criteria that required patients to be high risk or ineligible for anticoagulation, despite which 55% were on anticoagulation at 1 year. This finding may suggest a concern regarding clot formation outside the LAA or in any residual stump.

The main findings from the early registry studies of all three devices were stroke rates lower than predicted based on $CHADS_2$ score (which may have overestimated the anticipated stroke rate), significant risk of tamponade, and an important learning curve.

ASAP

Published trials as well as the commercial use of LAA closure devices other than the WATCHMAN device have largely enrolled patients with contraindications to anticoagulation, although the evidence base for placing these devices safely without anticoagulation is meager. The ASAP study (ASA Plavix Feasibility Study with WATCHMAN Left Atrial Appendage Closure Technology) was a multicenter prospective nonrandomized trial of 150 patients with contraindications to anticoagulation. The mean $CHADS_2$ score was 2.8 ± 1.2, thus higher than in most of the LAA closure device studies in the existing literature. Patients were treated with dual antiplatelet therapy; success rate was 94.7%. There were 2 tamponades (1.3%), 3 effusions, 1 device thrombus with ischemic stroke, 2 bleeding episodes, and 2 device embolizations. Through 14.4 ± 8.6 months of follow-up, there were 3 ischemic strokes (1.7%) compared with a predicted risk of 7.3%. If the potential benefits on stroke reduction of clopidogrel are factored in to the predicted event rate, the results still compare favorably with the predicted stroke risk of 5.1% based on the ACTIVE A trial (Atrial Fibrillation Clopidogrel Trial with Irbesartan for Prevention of Vascular Events).[27] There was systematic 3-month and 12-month transesophageal echo follow-up, again with core laboratory analysis; 6 cases of device thrombus were noted, 1 of which was associated with a stroke at 11 months. Although this study does not substitute for a randomized comparison of antiplatelet therapy versus device closure, the outcomes are generally comparable with if not superior to those seen with WATCHMAN plus anticoagulation therapy in PROTECT AF, raising the question of whether or not oral anticoagulation is necessary or beneficial[12]; the numbers are too small to eliminate the possibility of a type II error.

PROTECT AF

PROTECT AF, by far the strongest evidence base among the LAA occlusion trials to date, was a pivotal, pre–market approval study,[28] designed for a noninferiority analysis with a 2:1 noninferiority margin; 59 sites enrolled 707 patients (**Fig. 1**). Patients were randomized 2:1 to the WATCHMAN device or warfarin; those treated with the device had anticoagulation for a minimum of 45 days, with discontinuation if the LAA was adequately sealed. The study compared warfarin-eligible patients with a mean $CHADS_2$ score of 2.2 ± 1.1. Successful device placement occurred in 88%. The primary efficacy end point consisted of a composite of stroke, systemic embolism, and cardiovascular death.

PROTECT AF achieved its predefined end point (see **Fig. 1**A). There was reduction in primary efficacy end point results for the device compared with the warfarin group: at 1065 patient-years, there were 3.0 events per 100 patient-years in the device group versus 4.9 per 100 patient-years in the warfarin group, resulting in a noninferiority probability of more than 99.9%. As would be expected, hemorrhagic strokes occurred disproportionately in the warfarin group (1.6 per 100 patient-years vs 0.1 in the device group). However, there were an excess number of safety events in the patients randomized to WATCHMAN: 7.4 versus 4.4 per 100 patient-years (see **Fig. 1**B). The 2 most important procedure-related complications were pericardial tamponade rates of 5.0% and procedure-related stroke of 1.1%, the latter largely caused by air embolization. The systematic transesophageal echocardiographic follow-up (45 days, 6 months, and 1 year) showed 20 cases of device-associated thrombus (4.2%), although only 3 had associated strokes, an annualized rate of 0.3%.[12]

In a per protocol analysis examining the results after successful device placement and warfarin discontinuation in the device group, there was a statistically significant 60% reduction in the primary efficacy end point. Thus, the per protocol analysis provides a proof of concept that tends to confirm the overall hypothesis that exclusion of the LAA significantly reduces stroke, systemic embolism, and cardiovascular death.

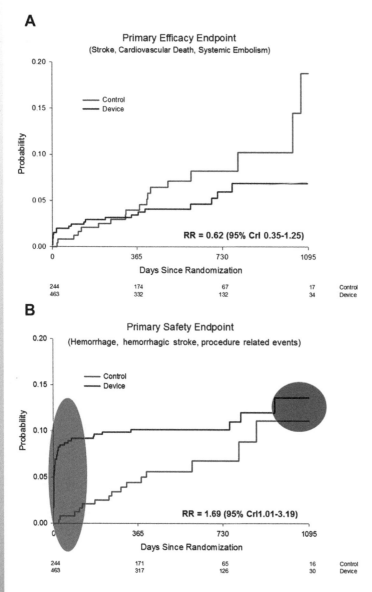

Fig. 1. Kaplan-Meier curve of primary efficacy (*A*) and primary safety (*B*) in the PROTECT AF trial. Patients randomized to warfarin represent the control group. The orange circle highlights the disproportionate safety event rates in patients undergoing WATCHMAN device placement in the immediate peri-implant period. The blue circle highlights the relative plateauing of events in the device group and the continued occurrence of adverse events, including bleeding, in the group on anticoagulation, so that the event rates approach (but do not cross). Crl, credibility interval; RR, relative risk. (*Adapted from* Holmes DR, Reddy VY, Turi ZG, et al. Percutaneous closure of the left atrial appendage versus warfarin therapy for prevention of stroke in patients with atrial fibrillation: a randomised non-inferiority trial. Lancet 2009; 374:538; with permission.)

A subsequent 2.3-year follow-up study[29] of PROTECT AF, encompassing 1588 patient-years, showed that 93.2% of WATCHMAN assigned patients successfully discontinued warfarin by 1 year. Anticoagulation was continued because of peridevice leak in 7.5%, 3.6% and 2.7% at 45 days, 6 months, and 1 year. The relationship of primary efficacy was 3.0% per year in the device group versus 4.3% per year in the patients randomized to anticoagulation; the safety event rates, although less dramatic in disparity than in the initial analysis, were 5.5% per year versus 3.6% for the warfarin group.

Criticisms of PROTECT AF were largely summarized in an editorial in the *New England Journal of Medicine* by Maisel,[30] the chairman of the US Food and Drug Administration (FDA) advisory panel that heard the initial presentation for device approval. Unusually, this editorial prepublished the results of the study itself. The criticisms can be summed up as: (1) sample size too small, (2) CHADS$_2$ score too low, (3) device group anticoagulation too much, (4) control group anticoagulation not enough, (5) learning curve too long, (6) complication rate too high, and (7) duration of follow-up too short. (8) The efficacy estimate rate was said to lack precision because of the wide relative risk confidence intervals inherent in the sample size and patient-years of follow-up.

To at least partially address the criticisms the following explanations have been offered: (1) although the sample size was smaller than trials of anticoagulants in atrial fibrillation, it was highly comparable with percutaneous cardiac device trials: coronary stenting (n = 410),[31] transcatheter aortic valve replacement (n = 1,040),[32,33] and percutaneous mitral valve repair (n = 957).[34] Moreover, adding the sample sizes of PROTECT AF, CAP (Continued Access Protocol), and PREVAIL, there were 1574 patients enrolled. (2) The CHADS$_2$ scores were low: 31% of the patients had a score of 1 in PROTECT AF, but the remaining 69% had essentially identical outcomes. (3) The fact that patients who could not take anticoagulation were excluded is a legitimate criticism, only partly addressed by the ASAP trial. However, this study design is largely mandated; the pivotal trial of the ACP was designed to enroll a similar population, with anticoagulation given to the device group for a similar period as in PROTECT AF. (4) The control group had a time in therapeutic range for anticoagulation of 66%, one of the highest rates in any warfarin anticoagulation study. (5) The learning curve was clearly an issue in PROTECT AF, but in PREVAIL, with improved training techniques and education, the tamponade rate was 1% among new operators versus 1.8% among experienced ones, and overall there was no difference between new and experienced operators in complications. (6) The complication rate in CAP and PREVAIL was substantially lower than in PROTECT AF, and (7) the duration of follow-up at 5 years is substantially higher than any other LAA occlusion technology. (8) The confidence intervals have narrowed substantially with 1500 patient-year follow-up,[29] and overall, the combined PROTECT AF and PREVAIL trials remain among the largest randomized clinical trials of a structural heart intervention device to date.

After enrollment in PROTECT AF was complete, a 460-patient CAP[12] showed a dramatic reduction in procedure-related or device-related safety events in the periprocedure period from 7.7% to 3.7%, with the rate of pericardial effusion requiring intervention decreasing from 5.0% to 2.2%. Procedure-related stroke declined from 0.9% to 0%. After a divided vote by an FDA panel in 2009, the agency elected not to approve device release, but rather mandated a follow-up trial, PREVAIL, which used a similar 2:1 randomization protocol, inclusion of new operators to document that the learning curve had been suitably addressed, and exclusion of patients with CHADS$_2$ scores of 1 eligible for aspirin-only therapy.

PREVAIL results are available on the Internet as an abstract presentation[9] intended for the 2013 American College of Cardiology Scientific Sessions (never presented because of an embargo violation); these results have not passed peer review and are discussed here in general terms. PREVAIL patients were generally older and had more comorbidities, as well as a higher CHADS$_2$ scores, than either PROTECT AF or the CAP trial. Implant success increased from 90.9% in PROTECT AF to 95.1% in PREVAIL. Two of the 3 primary end points in PREVAIL were met: (1) death, ischemic stroke, systemic embolism and procedure-related or device-related complications in the first 7 days were less than the performance goal mandated 2.62% upper bound (including 1.5% pericardial effusion and 0.4% cardiac perforation requiring repair), and (2) ischemic stroke or systemic embolism after the first 7 days was less than the 0.0275% upper bound. However, the warfarin group in PREVAIL had an extraordinarily low rate of stroke and systemic embolism: 0.7%; in comparison, none of the modern randomized studies of novel anticoagulants or PROTECT AF had a control group stroke or systemic embolism rate less than 1.5 per 100 patient-years. As a result, although the device group had a similarly low rate of stroke, systemic embolism, and cardiovascular death, this did not meet the prespecified noninferiority criterion. Neither PROTECT AF nor PREVAIL involved use of novel anticoagulants with their superior safety and efficacy profile, and thus our evidence base is derived solely from comparison with warfarin.

Controversy

The whole concept of LAA occlusion has been called into question. Concerns have been raised regarding the benefits of an intact LAA on homeostatic control of water, electrolytes, and adipose tissue. In an aggressive series of editorials, Stollberger and colleagues[35] proclaimed LAA occlusion to be a potential aggravating factor in the obesity epidemic as well as global warming. More grounded are concerns regarding potential peridevice leakage with both endovascular plugs as well as catheter-based and surgical pericardial and epicardial technologies, and thrombosis and embolism related both to leakage as well as residual stumps.

Procedural Complications

Each device has associated complications, some of which may look exaggerated, because most of the publications to date have incorporated operators' learning curves. Nevertheless, pericardial effusion has been a theme for each of the percutaneously implanted plugs. The LAA is a fragile structure[36] and a small effusion rate may be inevitable. Procedure-related pericardial effusion, discussed at length earlier, is likely inevitable in a small percentage, and has been ubiquitous in the overall left atrial intervention arena.[37] The pericardial effusion rate with LARIAT is primarily related to trauma to intrapericardial structures (eg, coronary arteries, chamber perforation) as well as trauma to the LAA; because a catheter is kept in the pericardium during the entire procedure and for some hours afterward, drainage is made relatively facile; lack of more than a rudimentary evidence base makes it uncertain if the effusion rate is understood.

Device embolization has been seen with all endocardially placed devices. Most data are available on the WATCHMAN device, with published data on 1152 patients, with an embolization rate of approximately 0.4%, an uncommon event in experienced hands.

The issue of residual leak after LAA closure has been a source of significant controversy. Lack of core laboratories, and variable definitions (and reporting) of peridevice leak, makes between-device comparisons impossible. Most information is available on the WATCHMAN device, in part because of systematic serial transesophageal echo follow-up. A series of 58 patients from a single site[38] reported leak in 34.5% of patients at 12 months, with growth in gap size over time. The issue was addressed in detail for the PROTECT AF study,[39] with a similar 32% of patients having peridevice flow at 12 months. However, in the larger cohort, the incidence decreased over time: 40.9% at 45 days and 33.8% at 6 months. Most peridevice leaks were moderate or major (1–3 mm and >3 mm, respectively), but there was no relationship between presence of peridevice flow and adverse events, nor did continuation of anticoagulation correlate with lower event rates. However, the analysis has a significant potential for type II error, and this issue requires continued analysis.

Residual leaks with the LARIAT device have been noted at the time of device placement,[24] as well as with leaks that seem to occur in follow-up.[40] Thrombus has been reported in a residual stump[41]; speculation has attributed other case reports to incomplete closure[42] or local inflammation induced by the epicardially placed snare.[43]

Percutaneous device closure of leaks has been reported with leaks associated with the LARIAT device and with surgery. Various devices have been used to close the leaks, including the ACP,[44] the Gore Septal Occluder,[45] and an Amplatzer Atrial Septal Occluder.[46]

Future Issues

The FDA Circulatory System Devices Panel meeting on December 11, 2013 resulted in a 13 to 1 vote in favor of approval of the WATCHMAN device. If the FDA approves device release, there will be significant issues regarding acceptable training to minimize the learning curve issues that were noted during PROTECT AF. There is a substantial need for a high-level evidence base with each of the percutaneous approaches and devices described, as well as in the surgical arena, including further evaluation of dedicated surgical LAA exclusion technologies.[47] Standardized definitions for efficacy and safety are needed.

The periprocedure and postprocedure polypharmacy needs further assessment. There is a need for comparison with newer anticoagulants in patients who are eligible, and for comparison with antiplatelet agents where those alone are tolerated. Both the ACP device and the LARIAT are touted as being appropriate for use without anticoagulation, and that issue has been inadequately addressed in both. The 2012 European Society Guidelines for the Management of Atrial Fibrillation,[48] assessing the existing evidence base, recommend LAA exclusion in patients with a high stroke risk and contraindication for long-term anticoagulation as class IIB (may be considered), level of evidence B (data derived from a single randomized clinical trial or large nonrandomized studies), citing only the PROTECT AF and subsequent Continued Access Registry. Ironically, the group for which the technology is being recommended (contraindications for anticoagulation) was not studied by these trials.

REFERENCES

1. Healey JS, Crystal E, Lamy A, et al. Left Atrial Appendage Occlusion Study (LAAOS): results of a randomized controlled pilot study of left atrial appendage occlusion during coronary bypass surgery in patients at risk for stroke. Am Heart J 2005; 150:288–93.
2. Glover RP, O'Neill TJ, Bailey CP. Commissurotomy for mitral stenosis. Circulation 1950;1:329–42.
3. Bolton HE, Delmonico JE Jr, Bailey CP. Prevention of cerebral embolism during mitral commissurotomy; results in 433 consecutive cases. Ann Intern Med 1954;41:272–81.
4. Ohtsuka T, Ninomiya M, Nonaka T, et al. Thoracoscopic stand-alone left atrial appendectomy for thromboembolism prevention in nonvalvular atrial fibrillation. J Am Coll Cardiol 2013;62:103–7.
5. Katz ES, Tsiamtsiouris T, Applebaum RM, et al. Surgical left atrial appendage ligation is frequently

incomplete: a transesophageal echocardiograhic study. J Am Coll Cardiol 2000;36:468–71.

6. Lynch M, Shanewise JS, Chang GL, et al. Recanalization of the left atrial appendage demonstrated by transesophageal echocardiography. Ann Thorac Surg 1997;63:1774–5.

7. Kanderian AS, Gillinov AM, Pettersson GB, et al. Success of surgical left atrial appendage closure: assessment by transesophageal echocardiography. J Am Coll Cardiol 2008;52:924–9.

8. Holmes DR, Reddy VY, Turi ZG, et al. Percutaneous closure of the left atrial appendage versus warfarin therapy for prevention of stroke in patients with atrial fibrillation: a randomised non-inferiority trial. Lancet 2009;374:534–42.

9. Holmes DR Jr. Randomized trial of LAA closure vs warfarin for stroke/thromboembolic prevention in patients with non-valvular atrial fibrillation (PREVAIL). American College of Cardiology. Available at: http://afibprofessional.cardiosource.org/~/media/Files/Science%20and%20Quality/Clinical%20Trials/ACC%2013%20Slides/PREVAIL%20Presentation%20Slides.ashx. Accessed March 5, 2014.

10. Block PC, Burstein S, Casale PN, et al. Percutaneous left atrial appendage occlusion for patients in atrial fibrillation suboptimal for warfarin therapy: 5-year results of the PLAATO (Percutaneous Left Atrial Appendage Transcatheter Occlusion) Study. JACC Cardiovasc Interv 2009;2:594–600.

11. Reddy VY, Mobius-Winkler S, Miller MA, et al. Left atrial appendage closure with the WATCHMAN device in patients with a contraindication for oral anticoagulation: the ASAP study (ASA Plavix Feasibility Study With WATCHMAN Left Atrial Appendage Closure Technology). J Am Coll Cardiol 2013;61:2551–6.

12. Reddy VY, Holmes D, Doshi SK, et al. Safety of percutaneous left atrial appendage closure: results from the WATCHMAN Left Atrial Appendage System for Embolic Protection in Patients with AF (PROTECT AF) clinical trial and the Continued Access Registry. Circulation 2011;123:417–24.

13. Gage BF, Waterman AD, Shannon W, et al. Validation of clinical classification schemes for predicting stroke: results from the National Registry of Atrial Fibrillation. JAMA 2001;285:2864–70.

14. Nakai T, Lesh MD, Gerstenfeld EP, et al. Percutaneous left atrial appendage occlusion (PLAATO) for preventing cardioembolism: first experience in canine model. Circulation 2002;105:2217–22.

15. Sick PB, Schuler G, Hauptmann KE, et al. Initial worldwide experience with the WATCHMAN left atrial appendage system for stroke prevention in atrial fibrillation. J Am Coll Cardiol 2007;49:1490–5.

16. Meier B, Palacios I, Windecker S, et al. Transcatheter left atrial appendage occlusion with Amplatzer devices to obviate anticoagulation in patients with atrial fibrillation. Catheter Cardiovasc Interv 2003;60:417–22.

17. Ostermayer SH, Reisman M, Kramer PH, et al. Percutaneous left atrial appendage transcatheter occlusion (PLAATO system) to prevent stroke in high-risk patients with non-rheumatic atrial fibrillation: results from the international multi-center feasibility trials. J Am Coll Cardiol 2005;46:9–14.

18. Park JW, Bethencourt A, Sievert H, et al. Left atrial appendage closure with Amplatzer cardiac plug in atrial fibrillation: initial European experience. Catheter Cardiovasc Interv 2011;77:700–6.

19. Sievert H, Lesh MD, Trepels T, et al. Percutaneous left atrial appendage transcatheter occlusion to prevent stroke in high-risk patients with atrial fibrillation: early clinical experience. Circulation 2002;105:1887–9.

20. Park JW, Leithauser B, Gerk U, et al. Percutaneous left atrial appendage transcatheter occlusion (PLAATO) for stroke prevention in atrial fibrillation: 2-year outcomes. J Invasive Cardiol 2009;21:446–50.

21. Bayard YL, Omran H, Neuzil P, et al. PLAATO (Percutaneous Left Atrial Appendage Transcatheter Occlusion) for prevention of cardioembolic stroke in non-anticoagulation eligible atrial fibrillation patients: results from the European PLAATO study. EuroIntervention 2010;6:220–6.

22. Sick PB, Yakubov SJ, Turi ZG, et al. Stroke prevention in non-valvular atrial fibrillation: long-term results of the WATCHMAN left atrial appendage occlusion pilot study (abstr). Eur Heart J 2009;30:599.

23. Urena M, Rodes-Cabau J, Freixa X, et al. Percutaneous left atrial appendage closure with the Amplatzer cardiac plug device in patients with nonvalvular atrial fibrillation and contraindications to anticoagulation therapy. J Am Coll Cardiol 2013;62:96–102.

24. Bartus K, Han FT, Bednarek J, et al. Percutaneous left atrial appendage suture ligation using the LARIAT device in patients with atrial fibrillation: initial clinical experience. J Am Coll Cardiol 2013;62:108–18.

25. Stone D, Byrne T, Pershad A. Early results with the LARIAT device for left atrial appendage exclusion in patients with atrial fibrillation at high risk for stroke and anticoagulation. Catheter Cardiovasc Interv 2013. [Epub ahead of print].

26. Turi ZG. The assault on the left atrial appendage in perspective. J Am Coll Cardiol 2013;62:119–20.

27. Connolly SJ, Pogue J, Hart RG, et al. Effect of clopidogrel added to aspirin in patients with atrial fibrillation. N Engl J Med 2009;360:2066–78.

28. Fountain RB, Holmes DR, Chandrasekaran K, et al. The PROTECT AF (WATCHMAN Left Atrial Appendage System for Embolic Protection in Patients with Atrial Fibrillation) trial. Am Heart J 2006;151:956–61.

29. Reddy VY, Doshi SK, Sievert H, et al. Percutaneous left atrial appendage closure for stroke prophylaxis in patients with atrial fibrillation: 2.3-year follow-up of the PROTECT AF (WATCHMAN Left Atrial Appendage System for Embolic Protection in Patients with Atrial Fibrillation) Trial. Circulation 2013; 127:720–9.

30. Maisel WH. Left atrial appendage occlusion – closure or just the beginning? N Engl J Med 2009; 360(25):2601–3.

31. Fischman DL, Leon MB, Baim DS, et al. A randomized comparison of coronary-stent placement and balloon angioplasty in the treatment of coronary artery disease. Stent Restenosis Study Investigators [see comments]. N Engl J Med 1994; 331:496–501.

32. Smith CR, Leon MB, Mack MJ, et al. Transcatheter versus surgical aortic-valve replacement in high-risk patients. N Engl J Med 2011;364:2187–98.

33. Leon MB, Smith CR, Mack M, et al. Transcatheter aortic-valve implantation for aortic stenosis in patients who cannot undergo surgery. N Engl J Med 2010;363:1597–607.

34. Feldman T, Foster E, Glower DD, et al. Percutaneous repair or surgery for mitral regurgitation. N Engl J Med 2011;364:1395–406.

35. Stollberger C, Finsterer J, Schneider B. Arguments against left atrial appendage occlusion for stroke prevention. Stroke 2007;38:e77.

36. Su P, McCarthy KP, Ho SY. Occluding the left atrial appendage: anatomical considerations. Heart 2008; 94:1166–70.

37. Holmes DR Jr, Nishimura R, Fountain R, et al. Iatrogenic pericardial effusion and tamponade in the percutaneous intracardiac intervention era. JACC Cardiovasc Interv 2009;2:705–17.

38. Bai R, Horton RP, Di BL, et al. Intraprocedural and long-term incomplete occlusion of the left atrial appendage following placement of the WATCHMAN device: a single center experience. J Cardiovasc Electrophysiol 2012;23:455–61.

39. Viles-Gonzalez JF, Kar S, Douglas P, et al. The clinical impact of incomplete left atrial appendage closure with the WATCHMAN device in patients with atrial fibrillation: a PROTECT AF (Percutaneous Closure of the Left Atrial Appendage Versus Warfarin Therapy for Prevention of Stroke in Patients With Atrial Fibrillation) substudy. J Am Coll Cardiol 2012;59:923–9.

40. Di Biase L, Burkhardt JD, Gibson DN, et al. 2D and 3D TEE evaluation of an early reopening of the LARIAT epicardial left atrial appendage closure device. Heart Rhythm 2013. [Epub ahead of print].

41. Briceno DF, Fernando RR, Laing ST. Left atrial appendage thrombus post LARIAT closure device. Heart Rhythm 2013. [Epub ahead of print].

42. Baker MS, Paul MJ, Gehi AK, et al. Left atrial thrombus after appendage ligation with LARIAT. Heart Rhythm 2013. [Epub ahead of print].

43. Giedrimas E, Lin AC, Knight BP. Left atrial thrombus after appendage closure using LARIAT. Circ Arrhythm Electrophysiol 2013;6:e52–3.

44. Mosley WJ, Smith MR, Price MJ. Percutaneous management of late leak after LARIAT transcatheter ligation of the left atrial appendage in patients with atrial fibrillation at high risk for stroke. Catheter Cardiovasc Interv 2013. [Epub ahead of print].

45. Matsumoto T, Nakamura M, Yeow WL, et al. Transcatheter left atrial appendage closure after incomplete surgical ligation. JACC Cardiovasc Interv 2013;6:e11–2.

46. Yeow WL, Matsumoto T, Kar S. Successful closure of residual leak following LARIAT procedure in a patient with high risk of stroke and hemorrhage. Catheter Cardiovasc Interv 2013. [Epub ahead of print].

47. Ailawadi G, Gerdisch MW, Harvey RL, et al. Exclusion of the left atrial appendage with a novel device: early results of a multicenter trial. J Thorac Cardiovasc Surg 2011;142:1002–9, 1009.e1.

48. Camm AJ, Lip GY, De CR, et al. 2012 focused update of the ESC Guidelines for the management of atrial fibrillation: an update of the 2010 ESC Guidelines for the management of atrial fibrillation. Developed with the special contribution of the European Heart Rhythm Association. Eur Heart J 2012;33: 2719–47.

Prevention and Management of Complications of Left Atrial Appendage Closure Devices

Matthew J. Price, MD

KEYWORDS

- Left atrial appendage • Atrial fibrillation • WATCHMAN device • Amplatzer cardiac plug • LARIAT
- Pericardial effusion

KEY POINTS

- The most common complication of left atrial appendage (LAA) occlusion or ligation is pericardial effusion, which may be caused during transseptal puncture, manipulation of equipment within the LAA, device deployment and retrieval, and, particular to the LARIAT procedure, dry pericardial access and manipulation of the endocardial and epicardial magnet-tipped wires.
- The incidence of periprocedural complications seems to decrease with increasing operator experience.
- Strategies to reduce the incidence of procedural complications include multiplanar imaging by 3-dimensional (3D) transesophageal echocardiography during transseptal puncture, use of a pigtail catheter to advance device delivery sheaths into the LAA, careful flushing of all left atrial sheaths, and avoidance of substantial tension on the epicardial wire during the LARIAT procedure.
- Awareness of, and preparation for, the management of procedural complications can increase patient safety and improve the risk-benefit ratio for LAA closure.

INTRODUCTION

Atrial fibrillation (AF) is associated with an ongoing risk of thromboembolic stroke and systemic embolism due to stasis and thrombus formation within the LAA. The risk of thromboembolic stroke and systemic embolism is estimated for a particular individual by incorporating comorbidities into risk scores such as the $CHADS_2$ and the CHA_2DS_2VASC models.[1–3] Warfarin, the oral direct factor Xa inhibitors rivoraxaban and apixaban, and the oral direct thrombin inhibitor dabigatran have been shown in large, randomized, clinical trials to reduce the risk of stroke but at the cost of major bleeding.[4–6] The decision to treat a patient with AF with anticoagulation is based on balancing these well-quantified thromboembolic and bleeding risks. Transcatheter LAA occlusion or ligation, by eliminating the nidus for thrombus formation, may reduce the thromboembolic risk in AF while abrogating the need for long-term anticoagulation and thereby eliminating the long-term bleeding risk observed with medical therapy. Device therapy, however, exposes the patient to a new hazard, that of procedural risk. The overall success of any effective device therapy depends critically on procedural safety, particularly when the goal of the device is to reduce the risk of a low-frequency event in an asymptomatic patient, such as LAA appendage closure for stroke prevention in AF. The issue of procedural safety is also of particular importance in the setting of LAA closure,

Disclosures: Dr M.J. Price reports receiving consulting fees from Boston Scientific, St. Jude, and Janssen Pharmaceuticals; research support (to institution) from SentreHeart; and honoraria for proctoring from SentreHeart.
Division of Cardiovascular Diseases, Scripps Clinic, 10666 North Torrey Pines Road, Maildrop S1056, La Jolla, CA 92037, USA
E-mail address: price.matthew@scrippshealth.org

Intervent Cardiol Clin 3 (2014) 301–311
http://dx.doi.org/10.1016/j.iccl.2013.12.001

as there exist minimal robust randomized clinical trial data to support its use compared with that supporting the use of oral anticoagulant therapy. Herein, the author reviews the available data pertaining to procedural risk during LAA closure, identifies common procedural complications, and discusses strategies for their prevention and management.

INCIDENCE OF COMPLICATIONS DURING TRANSCATHETER LAA CLOSURE
WATCHMAN LAA Occluder

The WATCHMAN LAA occluder (Boston Scientific, Natwick, MA, USA) consists of a nitinol frame and polyethylene terephthalate cap. Tines along the circumference of the midbody secure the device within the LAA after implantation. The device is introduced into the LAA through a 14F sheath delivered from the right femoral vein via a transseptal puncture. The appropriate-sized device is chosen through a combination of transesophageal echocardiography and fluoroscopy. Key procedural aspects that influence complication rates include transseptal technique, flushing of the large delivery sheath, manipulation of the delivery sheath and implantation of the device within the fragile and thin-walled LAA, and recognition of inappropriate device size or position (**Table 1**).

Procedural outcomes of WATCHMAN LAA occluder implantation have been examined in 2 randomized clinical trials performed in the United States,[7,8] a continuing access registry in the United States,[9] and 1 observational, European multicenter registry.[10] In the PROTECT-AF (WATCHMAN Left Atrial Appendage System for Embolic Protection in Patients with Atrial Fibrillation) trial, 463 patients were randomly allocated to device implantation; implantation was attempted in 449 patients. Serious pericardial effusion (requiring drainage or surgical intervention) occurred in 22 patients (4.8%) and nonserious pericardial effusions (requiring no intervention) occurred in an additional 8 patients (1.7%); procedure-related ischemic stroke occurred in 5 patients (1.1%), predominantly due to air embolism; cardiac perforation requiring surgical repair occurred in 7 patients (1.6%); and device embolization occurred in 3 patients (0.6%). Procedural outcomes seem to have improved since this initial experience: among the 460 patients enrolled within the Continuing Access to PROTECT-AF (CAP) registry, serious pericardial effusion within 7 days occurred in only 2.2% ($P = .019$ compared with PROTECT-AF), and there was only a single cardiac perforation requiring repair. With respect to the timing of complications, 89% of the serious pericardial effusions within PROTECT-AF and CAP were detected within 24 hours of the procedure. In PROTECT-AF, the cause of pericardial effusion was the transseptal puncture in 9% of cases; from manipulation within the LAA of sheaths, wires, catheters, or the delivery system in 41%; from the device deployment process in 18%; and from an unclear cause in 32%.[9] The subsequent PREVAIL (Prospective Randomized Evaluation of the WATCHMAN LAA Closure Device In Patients with Atrial Fibrillation Versus Long-Term Warfarin Therapy) randomized clinical trial further confirmed improved procedural safety, with rates of serious pericardial effusion similar to that of the CAP registry (1.5%); only 1 patient required surgical repair of a cardiac perforation.[8] Newer operators had similar procedural safety outcomes than experienced operators, suggesting that a substantial learning curve may not be required to achieve a safe result. Safety event rates in the smaller European ASAP (ASA Plavix Feasibility Study with WATCHMAN Left Atrial Appendage Closure Technology) registry were generally similar to that observed in CAP registry and PREVAIL. The improvement in procedural safety is likely due to changes in delivery sheath management, as detailed later.

Amplatzer Cardiac Plug

The Amplatzer cardiac plug (ACP) (St Jude Medical, Minneapolis, MN, USA), like the WATCHMAN LAA occluder, is a nitinol-based device that is implanted through a delivery sheath that is manipulated into the LAA via a transseptal puncture. Not surprisingly, similar types of procedural complications can occur, and, like the WATCHMAN experience, procedural safety has improved with time. In the original observational, European experience of 143 cases, the rate of tamponade was 4%, procedural stroke 2%, and device embolization 1%.[11] In a subsequent prospective, observational, adjudicated European multicenter registry of 204 patients undergoing ACP implantation, serious pericardial effusion occurred in 3 patients (1.5%), all of which occurred early; there were no procedure-related strokes; and there were 3 cases of device embolization (1.5%), all of which occurred within the first 7 days of implantation. A newer-generation ACP device incorporates design changes that may reduce the risk of embolization.[12] In summary, the procedural complications rates observed with the ACP are qualitatively similar to that seen with the WATCHMAN LAA occlude. The results of the ongoing Amplatzer Cardiac Plug randomized, clinical trial (NCT01118299) will provide further insights regarding device and procedural safety.

Table 1
Major procedural complications of left atrial appendage occluder implantation and potential preventive strategies

Complication	Cause	Preventative Strategy
Pericardial effusion	Initial transseptal puncture	TEE guidance (eg, X-plane) Avoid severe tenting of IAS
	Guidewire or catheter into LAA after initial transseptal puncture	Advance dilator into LAA under fluoroscopy over 0.32-in wire with distal curve or coronary wire
	Manipulation of delivery sheath/ system into and within LAA	Advance delivery sheath into LAA over pigtail catheter rather than guidewire
	Device deployment and retrieval	Maintain delivery sheath position; minimize retrievals and reimplantations if possible
Procedural stroke	Preexisting thrombus in LAA Insufficient anticoagulation	Careful baseline TEE Monitor anticoagulation, if possible; consider anticoagulation before transseptal puncture
	Air embolus from delivery sheath/ system	Flush sheath only after entering LAA and after device exchange, if performed
Device embolization	Inappropriate size	Tug-test; confirm device compression or appropriate fluoroscopic appearance
	Inappropriate position	Confirm device position and seal by TEE and fluoroscopy
Vascular (hematoma, arteriovenous fistula, pseudoaneurysm, bleeding)	Venous access	Careful technique; consider ultrasound guidance as needed

Abbreviation: TEE, transesophageal echocardiography.

Transcatheter Ligation of the LAA

Percutaneous ligation of the LAA is achieved using a combined subxiphoid and transseptal approach in which an epicardial suture is delivered with the LARIAT device (SentreHeart, Redwood City, CA, USA).[13] Potential complications may arise from transseptal access and delivery of equipment into the LAA. Other complications may arise from accessing the dry pericardium, deleterious interactions between the magnet-tipped wires that connect from within the LAA and the pericardial space, and the advancement and removal of the LARIAT device itself. Current understanding of real-world complication rates with the LARIAT procedure is limited to reports from a few single-center, observational studies. Bartus and colleagues[13] reported the results of 89 patients undergoing attempted transcatheter LAA ligation with the LARIAT device. Procedural complications occurred in 3 patients (3.3%): in one patient, there was a right ventricular perforation during pericardial access leading to hemopericardium that subsequently required drainage; one patient suffered

an epigastric artery laceration due to pericardial access; and a third patient had cardiac tamponade attributable to transseptal puncture. LAA perforation, hemothorax, and pleural effusions have also been reported in other experiences.[14,15]

STRATEGIES TO PREVENT COMPLICATIONS
Transseptal Puncture

Although the rates of major procedural complications are infrequent for transcatheter LAA occlusion or ligation, issues with transseptal access are a common underlying cause. Therefore, approaches that maximize the safety of this aspect of the procedure are critical for success. Several excellent reviews of transseptal techniques are available in the literature.[16] The transseptal puncture procedure is categorized into 5 phases: (1) evaluation of the LAA for preexisting thrombus, (2) tenting of the interatrial septum with the transseptal sheath dilator, (3) advancement of the transseptal needle through the interatrial septum, (4) passage of the transseptal sheath dilator and sheath into the left atrium, and

(5) removal of the dilator and flushing of the transseptal sheath. Complications may arise during each of these phases; the spectrum of complications that have been observed with transseptal puncture is listed in **Box 1**.

Evaluation of the LAA

Preprocedural transesophageal echocardiography (TEE) is required to ensure that there is no preexisting thrombus in the LAA before transseptal puncture and the delivery of equipment into the left atrium and LAA, as this could dislodge thrombus, resulting in a stroke or systemic embolization. A good rule of thumb is to defer the procedure if one would not perform a cardioversion in the setting of a similar-appearing LAA. The increased margin of safety provided by TEE or intracardiac echocardiography (ICE) guidance during needle puncture has led some operators to perform transseptal puncture in the presence of systemic anticoagulation, which may reduce the incidence of spontaneous thrombus formation in the LAA before the procedure, as well as reduce the possibility of thrombus formation on equipment within the LAA during the early stages of the procedure.

Entry of needle and transseptal sheath into the left atrium

Although transseptal puncture can be achieved safely with fluoroscopic guidance alone, ICE and TEE allow for the accurate positioning of the puncture for LAA occlusion/ligation and also provide visual clues that allow the operator to avoid catastrophic complications. Therefore, such guidance should be considered mandatory for transseptal puncture during LAA procedures, and possibly for all procedures that require transseptal puncture. The tenting of the interatrial septum with the dilator should be clearly visualized before advancement of the needle, preferably with 3D TEE X-plane, which can clearly indicate the superior/inferior and anterior/posterior location of the needle path through simultaneous imaging of the bicaval and aortic valve short axis views (**Fig. 1**). Tenting of the interatrial septum toward the aorta (and therefore risking aortic puncture) can be rectified by clockwise rotation of the needle/dilator/sheath system, and tenting directed posteriorly toward the left atrial free wall can be corrected with counterclockwise rotation. The needle should never be advanced if tenting is not clearly seen. Use of TEE can guide transseptal puncture even in the presence of substantial lipomatous hypertrophy of the interatrial septum or other complex septal anatomies (**Fig. 2**).

Substantial excursion of the interatrial septum despite advancement of the transseptal needle is an indicator that the needle has not crossed the septum and should be a warning of potential complications if care is not taken. Continued advancement of the transseptal system may lead to penetration of the back wall of the left atrium when the septum is finally crossed. Strategies to safely cross the septum in these circumstances include (1) advancement of the transseptal stylet or the stiff end of a coronary wire through the lumen of the transseptal needle under fluoroscopy just distal to the needle tip to puncture the septum and facilitate needle crossing or (2) use of radiofrequency energy with a dedicated transseptal needle (Baylis Medical, Montreal, QC, Canada) or application of high-frequency electric current to a conventional needle with a Bovie surgical blade (**Fig. 3**).

Once the interatrial septum appears to have been crossed by the needle, the operator can confirm this by several methods, including hemodynamics (ie, left atrial pressure measurement), contrast injection, observation of microcavitations in the left atrium after the application of radiofrequency energy, or advancement of a coronary wire deep into the left atrium or pulmonary vein. If there is any doubt that the needle may be in a different structure than the left atrium, the dilator should not be advanced; the needle should be withdrawn and transseptal puncture reattempted. Once the left atrial position is confirmed, the dilator can be advanced over the needle. A safe approach to advance the dilator is to advance it slightly over the needle; remove the needle, aspirate, and flush; and advance a 0.32-in wire with a broad curve at its tip through the dilator into the body of the left atrium or a standard 0.32-in J-tipped wire into

---

Box 1
Potential complications arising from transseptal puncture

Pericardial effusion and subsequent cardiac tamponade

Stroke

Myocardial ischemia/ST-T changes in the inferior leads

Persistence of atrial septal defect

Aortic root puncture

Puncture or tearing of right or left atrial free wall

Death

Data from Early MJ. How to perform a transseptal puncture. Heart 2009;95:85–92.

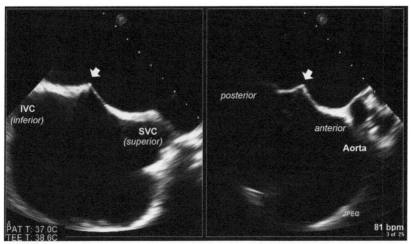

Fig. 1. Tenting of the interatrial septum on X-plane transesophageal echocardiography. The exact location of the transseptal puncture can be visualized by simultaneous imaging of the bicaval and aortic short axis planes. Clockwise rotation of the transseptal system provides a more posterior approach (visualized in the aortic short axis plane), whereas withdrawal of the system brings the puncture inferiorly (visualized in the bicaval plane). The degree of tenting can also be visualized, and excessive tenting despite forward pressure of the transseptal needle increases the risk of free-wall puncture after successful traversing of the interatrial septum by the needle; if this is visualized, alternative approaches, such as application of radiofrequency energy, may enable safe crossing. For left atrial appendage (LAA) occlusion or ligation, a posterior-inferior puncture is advantageous, as it allows for a coaxial approach for equipment to be introduced into the LAA. Arrows indicate tenting of interatrial septum by the transseptal sheath dilator. IVC, inferior vena cava; SVC, superior vena cava.

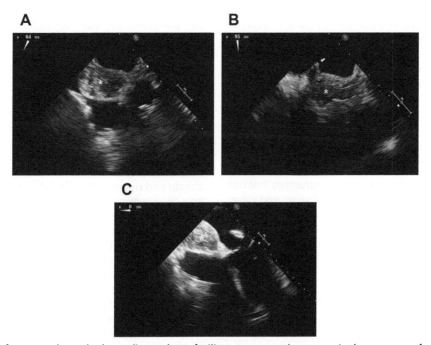

Fig. 2. Use of transesophageal echocardiography to facilitate transseptal puncture in the presence of marked lipomatous hypertrophy of the septum. A 77-year-old man with persistent atrial fibrillation and a high CHADS$_2$ score underwent left atrial appendage occlusion. (*A*) Transesophageal echocardiography (TEE) at the start of the procedure demonstrated a remarkably thick interatrial septum (*asterisk*). (*B*) Using TEE, the thin part of the interatrial septum (*asterisk*) was identified and the transseptal puncture was directed to this location, as evidenced by tenting (*arrow*). (*C*) TEE further demonstrated successful advancement of the transseptal sheath into the mid-left atrium.

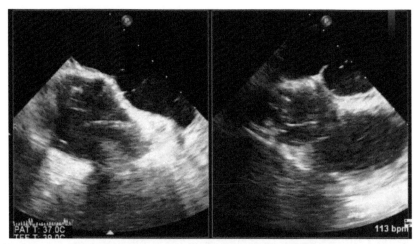

Fig. 3. Use of high frequency energy current to cross the interatrial septum. In this case, the transseptal needle could not cross the interatrial septum despite significant forward pressure and substantial excursion of the septum toward the left atrium. This situation could lead to puncture of the far wall of the atrium after crossing into the interatrial septum. Electrical energy was applied with an electrode (Bovie Medical Corporation, Clearwater, FL, USA) to a conventional transseptal needle that was gently pressed against the septum, and entry into the left atrium was confirmed by appearance of microcavitations in that chamber and the disappearance of tenting on echocardiography. Alternatively, a dedicated transseptal needle that delivers radiofrequency energy (Baylis Medical, Montreal, QC, Canada) can be used.

the left upper pulmonary vein (not the LAA) and advance the dilator and sheath over this wire. Alternatively, a coronary wire can be introduced into the needle, advanced into the pulmonary veins, the needle removed, and the dilator/sheath system safely advanced into the body of the left atrium.

Careful aspiration and flushing of the transseptal sheath after removing the dilator is critical. Maintaining the proximal end of the sheath below the level of the right atrium whenever the stopcock is manipulated can help prevent inadvertent introduction of air into the system, risking air embolism.

Introduction of Equipment into the Left Atrial Appendage

The LAA is a thin-walled, friable structure that can easily be torn or perforated by catheters and wires. All current techniques for transcatheter LAA occlusion or ligation require introduction of delivery equipment into the LAA. A large-caliber sheath must be introduced into the LAA in the case of the ACP and WATCHMAN devices, and a magnetic-tipped wire and over-the-wire balloon catheter must be advanced into the LAA in the case of the LARIAT procedure.

LAA occluder delivery sheaths

The tip of a guide or sheath can fairly easily rend the LAA wall. In the case of the WATCHMAN device, the delivery sheath must be introduced fairly deeply into the LAA and often rotated substantially to achieve a coaxial orientation between the

sheath and the LAA. A safe approach to sheath introduction consists of a telescoping technique. First, the delivery sheath is introduced into the left atrium over a stiff wire placed in the left upper pulmonary vein. If a guide wire cannot be placed into the pulmonary vein, the delivery sheath may be safely advanced over an Inoue wire (Toray Medical Company Ltd, Chiba, Japan) placed within the left atrium. Next, the wire is removed and the sheath is carefully aspirated and flushed. This step is critical, as air embolism has been a reported complication of WATCHMAN implantation,[7] likely due to insufficient flushing or attempted aspiration and flushing after introduction of the device into the delivery sheath. A 5F or 6F diagnostic pigtail catheter is advanced within the sheath and manipulated into an appropriate position deep within the LAA. The delivery sheath is then advanced over the pigtail catheter, which acts as a support rail and helps prevent the tip of the delivery sheath from contacting the LAA wall despite deep engagement (**Fig. 4**). The adoption of this telescoping approach, in addition to strict protocols for sheath flushing, may have contributed to the reduction in procedural complications noted in the latter half of the PROTECT-AF trial and the CAP registry,[9] as well as the PREVAIL trial.[8]

LAA management during the LARIAT procedure

The LARIAT procedure first requires introduction of the magnet-tipped EndoWire deep into the

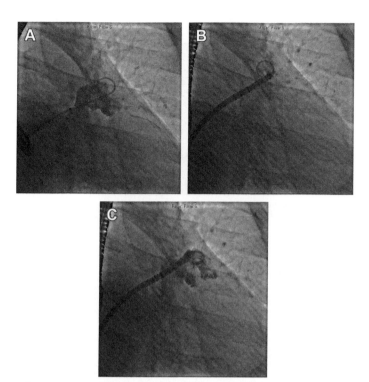

Fig. 4. Advancement of WATCHMAN delivery sheath using a telescoping system to prevent LAA injury from the sheath tip. (*A*) A 6F diagnostic pigtail catheter is advanced through the 14F delivery sheath deep into the LAA. (*B*) The pigtail catheter is fixed with one hand and the delivery sheath is advanced over the catheter deeper into the LAA. (*C*) The sheath is advanced further to the distal portion of the LAA together with counterclockwise rotation to achieve a coaxial position. Contrast injection through the pigtail catheter confirms the position.

anterior lobe of the LAA. A balloon catheter is then advanced over the EndoWire and is used to identify the LAA os on fluoroscopy. Although the tip of the EndoWire is floppy, the operator must recognize any resistance to advancement, as this usually denotes that the magnet tip is against the LAA wall. If the EndoWire is not in the appropriate place within the LAA, the wire should be withdrawn slightly and manipulated accordingly. The over-the-wire balloon catheter can act as a support catheter to negotiate entry into the various LAA lobes, but the operator must realize that the further distal the balloon catheter relative to the EndoWire (SentreHeart Inc, Redwood City, CA, USA), the stiffer the tip of the EndoWire becomes, increasing the risk of LAA perforation with aggressive manipulation of the EndoWire. This risk is especially the case with shallow or small LAAs when identifying the LAA os necessitates advancing the balloon catheter just proximal to the EndoWire magnet. It is also critical to recognize the danger of unintended tension on the EndoWire after connection with the magnet-tipped EpiWire. Unwanted traction on the EpiWire (SentreHeart Inc, Redwood City, CA, USA), which can occur during advancement or removal of the LARIAT loop, can pull the

EpiWire magnet through the LAA wall, leading to LAA perforation and subsequent pericardial effusion and tamponade (**Fig. 5**).

Device Embolization

A detailed description of the appropriate techniques to avoid LAA device embolization is beyond the scope of this article. In brief, the simple acronym "PASS" can be used by the operator as a final checklist before WATCHMAN device release: P for *position* on TEE and fluoroscopy; A for anchor, assessed through a tug-test S for sealed on TEE and fluoroscopy; and S for size, where on TEE the device should be 8–20% compressed. A similar set of principles can be applied to the ACP. Although the absolute incidence of device embolization is quite low in the reported experience of the WATCHMAN device and ACP, one advantage of transcatheter LAA ligation with the LARIAT device is the lack of such a potential complication because no device is left behind.

Pericardial Access Complications

The approach to dry pericardial access is addressed in other articles in this issue. In brief, the

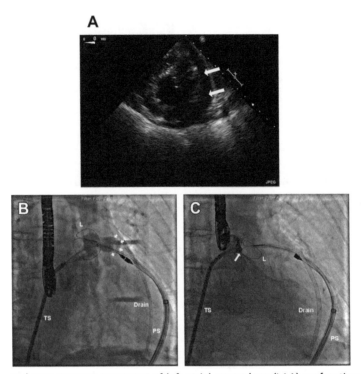

Fig. 5. Recognition and percutaneous treatment of left atrial appendage (LAA) perforation. (*A*) Accumulating pericardial effusion (*arrows*) was noted on transesophageal echocardiography after advancement of a LARIAT device over the endocardial-epicardial rail. (*B*) A pericardial drain was introduced and autotransfusion performed (stopcock and tubing connecting pericardial drain with femoral venous sheath); fluoroscopy also demonstrated that the EndoWire magnet tip was in the pericardium, outside of the border of the LAA (*arrows*: LAA border by LA angiography). The extracardiac position of the EndoWire was further confirmed by contrast injection through the lumen of the over-the-wire balloon catheter. (*C*) The pericardial drain was exchanged over a wire for a 9F sheath to increase the volume of blood that could be removed and autotransfused during reattempt and ultimately successful LARIAT closure (*arrow*, ligated LAA). After LARIAT deployment, there was no further accumulation of pericardial fluid and the postprocedural course was uneventful. L, LARIAT; PS, pericardial sheath; TS, transseptal sheath.

anterior approach provides a margin of safety because the anterior mediastinum is empty of vital structures. Challenging aspects that may increase the risk of complication include a narrow window between the sternum and right ventricular wall, which can be recognized on preprocedural computed tomography. Pericardial access is generally obtained before transseptal puncture and systemic anticoagulation. A 17-gauge, 150-mm Pajunk Tuohy needle (PAJUNK GmbH Medizintechnologie, Geisingen, Germany) is commonly used, as the upwardly directed bevel at the distal tip directs the needle away from the right ventricular wall (**Fig. 6**). A micropunture needle can also be used. After the needle is advanced under the sternum and directed downward toward the cardiac shadow, gentle injection of dilute contrast through the needle lumen in the left lateral projection demonstrates tenting of the parietal pericardium and helps visualize entry into the pericardial space after the

needle is advanced slightly further (**Fig. 7**). As dilators and the pericardial sheath are advanced into the pericardial space over a 0.35-in wire, the operator should confirm that TEE demonstrates no right ventricular compression. If compression is observed, repeat pericardial access at a different site should be considered.

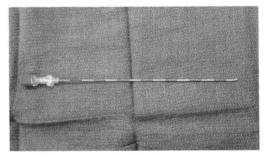

Fig. 6. A 17-gauge Pajunk Tuohy cannula commonly used for dry pericardial access.

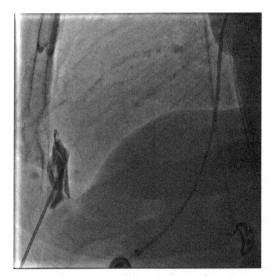

Fig. 7. Injection of dilute radiographic contrast through the Tuohy needle demonstrates tenting of the parietal pericardium. The needle was directed under the sternum toward approximately the 2-o'clock position in the anterior-posterior projection and then directed downward toward the cardiac shadow in the left lateral projection. After tenting was achieved, the needle was advanced further, and repeat contrast injection demonstrated filling of the pericardial space.

MANAGEMENT STRATEGIES
Pericardial Effusion

A thorough understanding and plan for the management of a significant pericardial effusion is critical for the operator as this is the most common complication observed with all the approaches to LAA closure. Placement of a second femoral venous sheath at the start of the procedure to serve as a "bailout" in case of hemodynamic compromise can be considered, unless the anesthesiologist has placed a jugular venous line. This second venous access is useful for fluid administration or for autotransfusion in the setting of massive pericardial hemorrhage, as described later. Evaluation for any baseline pericardial effusion and constant communication between the echocardiographer and the operator during the procedure regarding the status of the pericardial space can also help identify issues early before tamponade occurs. For slow-growing, stable effusions, standard pericardiocentesis followed by placement of a pericardial drain and reversal of heparin anticoagulation (if equipment is no longer in the left atrium) is usually adequate. Small LAA tears, lacerations, and perforations often close spontaneously if blood is aggressively removed from the pericardium.

Pericardial effusion or tamponade during the LARIAT procedure

The approach to the management of pericardial effusion that occurs during the LARIAT procedure is somewhat unique. If an effusion forms early after pericardial sheath introduction and before advancement of the other equipment into the pericardium, the fluid can be removed through the pericardial sheath itself. The pericardial sheath has no lumen for flushing or aspiration, but the sheath can be carefully exchanged for a standard, large-bore sheath or drain over a wire. Alternatively, the fluid can be removed with a diagnostic pigtail catheter that is simply advanced through the pericardial sheath. Placing a "bailout" 0.35-in wire alongside the pericardial sheath at the start of the procedure may be helpful for pericardial access if a significant effusion subsequently occurs. If the cause of the effusion is a perforation during manipulation of the LARIAT device over the LAA, a definitive solution is to quickly snare and exclude the LAA (see **Fig. 5**), often while simultaneously performing autotransfusion. Even if the LAA cannot be ligated successfully, tacking up the LAA by maintaining a dry pericardium with aggressive effusion removal for several minutes can seal the perforation.

Autotransfusion

Autotransfusion of blood aspirated from the pericardium enables the operator to maintain hemodynamic stability and attempt to seal the cardiac perforation despite substantial and persistent fluid accumulation. First, a pericardial drain or an 8F or 9F sheath is introduced into the pericardium. Second, another 6F to 8F sheath is introduced into the femoral vein (or was already placed as a bailout at the start of the procedure). The drain is connected to the venous sheath with a stopcock and male-to-male tubing (or an appropriate adapter if male-to-female tubing is used). Blood is aspirated from the drain using a large syringe and then pushed back into the venous system. This process is continued for several minutes until the pericardium is dry, which often stops the leak by allowing the perforation to seal. In the author's anecdotal experience, autotransfusion can be performed for as long as 20 to 30 minutes with eventual success. Continued autotransfusion should be aborted if aspiration of a rapidly reaccumulating effusion seems futile (eg, due to the length of time or impending hemodynamic compromise despite aggressive fluid removal). In this case, surgery is required (**Fig. 8**).

Chest Pain

Acute and prolonged chest discomfort has been observed after the LARIAT procedure. This

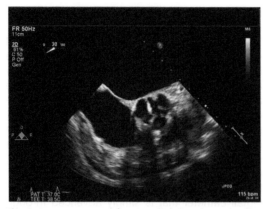

Fig. 8. Large amount of pericardial clot along the free wall of the right ventricle by TEE after prolonged pericardiocentesis and autotransfusion. In this case, a pericardial effusion formed soon after pericardial access, and the effusion persistently reoccurred despite prolonged autotransfusion. Furthermore, the pericardial clot could not be removed through aspiration. Hemodynamic stability could not be consistently maintained, and the patient went urgently to cardiac surgery, where the pericardial clot was evacuated, revealing a perforation at the apex of the right ventricle, which was easily repaired.

discomfort may be due to pericardial inflammation and/or necrosis of the LAA. Anecdotally, the early chest discomfort after the LARIAT procedure may in large part arise simply from the pericardial drain that is left in after the procedure (as it is within a dry pericardial space) and is relieved after drain removal. Some operators elect to remove the drain as early as 4 to 6 hours postprocedure as long as there is little ongoing drainage (eg, <25 mL/h). Other approaches to limit postprocedure pain include prophylactic ketorolac before or during the procedure in patients with normal renal function, intrapericardial administration of lidocaine at the end of the procedure, and a short course of oral colchicine. However, there are no data regarding the efficacy of any of these approaches. Corticosteroids should be avoided given the potential impact on healing and anecdotal reports of late leak (Dr Randall Lee, personal communication, 2013).

SUMMARY

Transcatheter occlusion or ligation of the LAA represents a paradigm shift in the prevention of stroke in patients with AF. However, because LAA occlusion or ligation is a preventative strategy, and large randomized trials have demonstrated the safety and efficacy of oral anticoagulants, minimizing the incidence of procedural complications is critical for the broad adoption of these technologies.

Furthermore, when complications occur, their management must limit long-term morbidity. Observational registries and randomized trials have demonstrated that pericardial effusion is the most common procedural complication irrespective of LAA occlusion technology. Transseptal puncture, manipulation of sheaths and other equipment in the LAA, device retrieval, and, in the case of the LARIAT device, dry pericardial access and Endo-Epicardial wire manipulation are key causes of pericardial effusions; heightened awareness and careful technique are required to avoid these complications and manage them safely. The incidence of procedural complications seems to decrease with increased communal experience. As such, the risk-benefit ratio of LAA occlusion and ligation will continue to improve, thereby providing a much-needed alternative to chronic anticoagulation in patients with AF who are at significant risk for thromboembolic events.

REFERENCES

1. Fuster V, Ryden LE, Cannom DS, et al. 2011 ACCF/ AHA/HRS Focused Updates Incorporated Into the ACC/AHA/ESC 2006 Guidelines for the Management of Patients With Atrial Fibrillation: A Report of the American College of Cardiology Foundation/ American Heart Association Task Force on Practice Guidelines Developed in partnership with the European Society of Cardiology and in collaboration with the European Heart Rhythm Association and the Heart Rhythm Society. J Am Coll Cardiol 2011; 57(11):e101–98.
2. Lip GY, Nieuwlaat R, Pisters R, et al. Refining clinical risk stratification for predicting stroke and thromboembolism in atrial fibrillation using a novel risk factor-based approach: the Euro Heart Survey on Atrial Fibrillation. Chest 2010;137(2):263–72.
3. Gage BF, Waterman AD, Shannon W, et al. Validation of clinical classification schemes for predicting stroke: results from the National Registry of Atrial Fibrillation. JAMA 2001;285(22):2864–70.
4. Connolly SJ, Ezekowitz MD, Yusuf S, et al. Dabigatran versus warfarin in patients with atrial fibrillation. N Engl J Med 2009;361(12):1139–51.
5. Patel MR, Mahaffey KW, Garg J, et al. Rivaroxaban versus warfarin in nonvalvular atrial fibrillation. N Engl J Med 2011;365(10):883–91.
6. Granger CB, Alexander JH, McMurray JJ, et al. Apixaban versus warfarin in patients with atrial fibrillation. N Engl J Med 2011;365(11):981–92.
7. Holmes DR, Reddy VY, Turi ZG, et al. Percutaneous closure of the left atrial appendage versus warfarin therapy for prevention of stroke in patients with atrial fibrillation: a randomised non-inferiority trial. Lancet 2009;374(9689):534–42.

8. Holmes D. Results of randomized trial of left atrial appendage closure versus warfarin for stroke/thromboembolic prevention in patients with non-valvular atrial fibrillation. American College of Cardiology Scientific Sessions. San Francisco (CA), March 9, 2013.

9. Reddy VY, Holmes D, Doshi SK, et al. Safety of percutaneous left atrial appendage closure: results from the Watchman Left Atrial Appendage System for Embolic Protection in Patients with AF (PROTECT AF) clinical trial and the Continued Access Registry. Circulation 2011;123(4): 417–24.

10. Reddy VY, Mobius-Winkler S, Miller MA, et al. Left atrial appendage closure with the Watchman device in patients with a contraindication for oral anticoagulation: The ASAP Study (ASA Plavix Feasibility Study with Watchman Left Atrial Appendage Closure Technology). J Am Coll Cardiol 2013;61(25):2551–6.

11. Park JW, Bethencourt A, Sievert H, et al. Left atrial appendage closure with Amplatzer cardiac plug in atrial fibrillation: initial European experience. Catheter Cardiovasc Interv 2011;77(5):700–6.

12. Freixa X, Chan JL, Tzikas A, et al. The Amplatzer Cardiac Plug 2 for left atrial appendage occlusion: novel features and first-in-man experience. EuroIntervention 2013;8(9):1094–8.

13. Bartus K, Han FT, Bednarek J, et al. Percutaneous left atrial appendage suture ligation using the LARIAT device in patients with atrial fibrillation: initial clinical experience. J Am Coll Cardiol 2012;62(2):108–18.

14. Shetty R, Leitner JP, Zhang M. Percutaneous catheter-based left atrial appendage ligation and management of periprocedural left atrial appendage perforation with the LARIAT suture delivery system. J Invasive Cardiol 2012;24(11):E289–93.

15. Stone D, Byrne T, Pershad A. Early results with the LARIAT device for left atrial appendage exclusion in patients with atrial fibrillation at high risk for stroke and anticoagulation. Catheter Cardiovasc Interv 2013. [Epub ahead of print].

16. Earley MJ. How to perform a transseptal puncture. Heart 2009;95(1):85–92.

Index

Note: Page numbers of article titles are in **boldface** type.

Moving?

Make sure your subscription moves with you!

To notify us of your new address, find your **Clinics Account Number** (located on your mailing label above your name), and contact customer service at:

Email: journalscustomerservice-usa@elsevier.com

800-654-2452 (subscribers in the U.S. & Canada)
314-447-8871 (subscribers outside of the U.S. & Canada)

Fax number: 314-447-8029

Elsevier Health Sciences Division
Subscription Customer Service
3251 Riverport Lane
Maryland Heights, MO 63043

*To ensure uninterrupted delivery of your subscription, please notify us at least 4 weeks in advance of move.

Printed and bound by CPI Group (UK) Ltd, Croydon, CR0 4YY

03/10/2024

01040375-0011